a guide to
headaches
& migraines

Katherine Wright

Published 2014 by Geddes & Grosset
an imprint of The Gresham Publishing Company Ltd.,
Academy Park, Building 4000, Gower Street, Glasgow, G51 1PR, Scotland

First published 2009. Repritned 2014.

ISBN 978 1 84205 650 9

Printed and bound in the EU

The material contained in this book is set out in good faith for general guidance
only. Whilst every effort has been made to ensure that the information in this
book is accurate, relevant and up to date, this book is sold on the condition that
neither the author nor the publisher can be found legally responsible for the
consequences of any errors or omissions.

Diagnosis and treatment are skilled undertakings which must always be carried
out by a doctor and not from the pages of a book.

CONTENTS

Chapter 9
A SUMMARY OF THE ENVIRONMENTAL AND
LIFESTYLE CAUSES OF HEADACHES

Chapter 10
EFFECTS OF HEADACHES AND MIGRAINES
ON EVERYDAY LIFE

Chapter 11
SECONDARY HEADACHES:
POSSIBLE CAUSES

Part One

HEADACHES AND MIGRAINES: SYMPTOMS, CAUSES AND TREATMENT

Chapter 1

INTRODUCTION

The experience of headache is universal among human beings, affecting people of both sexes from infancy until old age. It is also fascinating to note that scientists increasingly believe that other mammalian species have headaches as well. In people, some types of headache show a gender bias and it is also the case that the type of headache to which a person is subject tends to change with aging. Additionally, an individual may experience more than one type of headache during any particular time period. Hence a person who commonly has migraines may occasionally experience a headache of a different type.

Although around 150 different causes for headaches have been identified, doctors recognise relatively few types and these are the ones that most commonly affect the majority of people. Categorising headaches has always proved problematic and this is reflected in the fact that there is a degree of overlap between the medical terms and definitions used to describe them.

The experience of headache varies greatly, not only between individuals but also in the same person. It is possible for an individual to have an intense and painful headache on one occasion and one that is hardly noticeable the next time it occurs.

Some people experience headaches at night while others have headaches that are linked to already existing conditions such as thyroid disorders. Sometimes headaches are experienced in conjunction with other disorders such as epilepsy or because of actual injuries to the head.

It is acknowledged that there is a strong psychological component both in the generation and experience of certain types of headache but this is certainly not the same as saying that headaches are 'all in the mind'. However, the fact that this is the case means that there is a role not only for orthodox medicine but also for complementary therapies in the treatment, management and prevention of headaches and migraines and many of these are explored in part two of this book.

It is hoped that this guide will prove helpful not only to those who are often afflicted by headaches or migraines but also to those who simply wish to learn a little more. While every attempt has been made to provide accurate information, this book should not be used for self-diagnosis or treatment. As with all aspects of health, if you are experiencing headaches on a regular basis or are worried or concerned about your symptoms, it is always best to seek medical advice.

Chapter 2

DEFINITIONS AND TERMS: HEADACHE OR MIGRAINE?

Primary and secondary headaches

The generally accepted guidelines for the classification of headaches have been devised by an organisation called the International Headache Society. However, these criteria may not always be rigidly followed and may be open to differing interpretations and application by individual doctors.

The simplest and most basic classification of headaches defines them as either *primary* or *secondary*. *Primary* headaches arise spontaneously and they are by far the most common group, accounting for around 90% of all cases. *Secondary* headaches occur as a symptom of another underlying disorder or illness and since only about 10% of all cases fall into this category, they are evidently uncommon. However, although it is rare for any particular instance of a headache to be caused by a serious medical condition, with fewer than 5% of people who seek medical advice for headaches having any form of serious disorder as the cause of their symptoms, it is perhaps more helpful to clarify this a little by saying that with feverish, viral infections, such as the common cold or flu, a secondary headache is a frequent accompanying symptom and most people will experience this at some stage or another in their lifetime.

Acute and chronic headaches

Other terms that are commonly used to categorise headaches are *acute* (also, *acute single* or *episodic*) and *chronic* (also, *chronic daily* or *recurrent*). Difficulties arise with the use of all these terms, which can perhaps be most usefully thought of as a sort of sliding scale of definition.

An *acute headache* is one that arises as a single, one-off event or, at least, occurs rarely and in isolation over a generally lengthy time period. Hence a secondary headache of an unusual cause could be described as acute but equally, so can the very first experience of a primary headache that a person has, commonly during childhood.

Chronic headaches are strictly defined as ones that occur on at least 15 days of each month for a minimum period of 6 months. However, it is apparent that an over-rigid application of this definition might not always prove to be useful. Common sense suggests that anyone afflicted by headaches on a regular basis should be called a chronic sufferer, whether or not they fulfil these strict time criteria. Finally, the category of *chronic daily headaches* can be applied to any of the three *types* of headache described below, if these are occurring on at least 15 days of each month for 6 months or longer.

Types of primary headache

All the terms outlined above are fairly general in their application but the three main *types* of headache recognised by doctors are more tightly and specifically defined. All of them are primary in nature and they may be either acute or chronic, according to the frequency of their occurrence. However, it is probably safe to assert that if a headache of any type has become significant enough to be regarded as a problem then it is likely that it is happening on a regular basis, even though it may not be frequent enough to be classed as chronic according to the strict definition.

The three types of commonly occurring, primary headache, each of which is defined by a fairly specific set of symptoms are called *tension headaches*, *cluster headaches* and *migraine headaches* and these are considered in greater detail below.

Chapter 3
TENSION HEADACHES

What is a tension headache?

Tension headaches are the most frequently occurring type of primary headache, accounting for 70% of all instances and commonly experienced by most people at some stage in life. They may be given the alternative names of *stress headaches* or *muscular headaches*, and they can affect people of both sexes at any age, although they are less likely to arise in pre-adolescent children. This type of headache is associated with contraction (tension) of the muscles in the upper back and neck and produces a mild to moderate, generalised pain, rather than one which is localised at a particular point. It is common for the pain to be experienced as pressure around the circumference of the head, as though a band was being gradually tightened and the head squeezed. However, sometimes the pain is felt more at the back of the head and the person can be very much aware of the contraction and tightness of the neck muscles. The pain is constant rather than throbbing, although it may begin as mild discomfort and build gradually over several hours to a greater level of intensity. It is not made significantly worse by ordinary movements or routine physical activity although it may be exacerbated by intense levels of exercise. There is no accompanying nausea or vomiting and neither is there any heightened sensitivity to noise or light.

A tension headache usually occurs during the normal round of daily activity but exhaustion and worry can trigger a headache while you sleep or it may be present on first waking up in the morning. The pain is usually short-lived, lasting at most for a day, and is generally effectively relieved by common, over-the-counter analgesic medication.

Causes

Many people experience a tension headache at least once or twice a month while for others its occurrence is a rare event. It is not normally necessary to consult a doctor for an occasional occurrence of tension headache and there is nothing to be gained by doing so. It may or may not be possible to identify the cause or triggering factor for one particular headache and the person affected is best qualified to be the judge of this, rather than a doctor. The only useful purpose served is if it then becomes possible to avoid the trigger in the future and so hopefully avert a recurrence of the pain. For example, holding a phone between your ear and shoulder when busy at work can cause a tension headache and once identified as a trigger, it is easy enough to stop doing this. However, identifying the cause of a tension headache remains highly problematic for most people. This is because the most common cause or trigger of this type of headache is the kind of stress and anxiety that are practically universal in everyday life. These psychological factors, together with the internal biochemical changes that they provoke, are all held to play a part in the generation of a tension headache.

Even the most relaxed, unflurried person who believes himself to be impervious to stress will occasionally experience a tension headache. Equally, one individual's ability to cope with stress varies from one episode to another and hence, perhaps, the likelihood of experiencing a headache on any particular occasion. Although it is practically impossible to entirely avoid the stresses that may lead to a headache, there are ways to lessen or mitigate both the emotional and physical effects, such as the tightening of muscles. Many of the complementary therapies described later in Part Two of this book work precisely in this way. They are helpful in counteracting the effects of stress and as well as being of great use in this regard they also indirectly help to relieve headache pain itself.

Although it is often difficult to pinpoint the exact cause of any particular headache, certain other predisposing factors in addition to stress are recognised. Of these, two have been identified as important in relation to tension headaches: *eye-strain* and *poor posture*.

Eye-strain

Eye-strain is one well-known factor and in this context, it is usually refers to a struggle to read but could, of course, equally be connected with any close, concentrated work such as sewing or art and craft. It is surprisingly common for people to strain their eyes in this way, perhaps because they have not needed assistance in the past and simply do not realise that they now require reading glasses. Also, among those who do already wear glasses, it is common to fail to notice that the eyes have changed and that another check-up and new prescription is overdue.

It is recommended that all adults should have an eye test every three years and this is provided as a free service on the NHS. An eye test becomes increasingly important with age, since the close examination of the back of the eyes can diagnose other problems, such as glaucoma and hypertension, as well as identifying the gradual changes in focusing ability that naturally take place over time. At all ages in life, it is important to ensure that reading or close work is carried out in good light. Squinting or 'screwing up' the eyes causes contraction both of the brow muscles (hence frowning) and those of the scalp, and this tension can easily be relayed to the neck and upper spine. It can readily be appreciated how all this favours the production of a headache.

Eye-strain is not just confined to problems with reading the printed word but has become increasingly recognised as a risk connected with the widespread use of computer monitors and, perhaps, with mobile phones.

Poor posture

A further, well-recognised, predisposing factor is poor posture and this is something that may begin as early as adolescence. It is easy to understand how a rounding of the upper back and shoulders, coupled with incorrect head carriage, can result in tension in the muscles of the neck and upper spine. Postural problems have been particularly recognised as a risk factor for white collar, sedentary office workers – those who sit behind desks all day, increasingly, in recent years, using computers. Evidently in these circumstances, a combination of eye-strain and incorrect posture might be the cause of tension headaches.

A great deal of time and effort has been put into the design and production of office chairs that support the back and promote correct posture and these are now widely available. Also, the Health and Safety Executive (HSE) produce mandatory guidelines for employers aimed at safeguarding the health of office workers and these include regulations on the maximum length of time that should be spent in front of computer screens and the provision of eye tests.

Treatment

Tension headaches can usually be effectively treated by taking common, over-the-counter, pain-relieving remedies such as paracetamol, aspirin or ibuprofen. Codeine should be used with caution as overuse of this medicine can, in itself, be the cause of headaches. It is best to take the recommended dose as soon as the headache starts and possibly repeat the dose four hours later, should this prove to be necessary. Other simple measures may also be helpful, depending upon the severity of the headache. These include rest, relaxation and sleep, the application of a cold flannel to the forehead and gentle massage of the muscles of the neck, shoulders and scalp.

Prevention

It is probably impossible to entirely prevent the occurrence of tension headaches but for frequent sufferers, there are various strategies that can be tried. These include keeping a headache diary (*see* page 49), which may help to pinpoint any common patterns or triggers in the occurrence of the headaches. If triggers can be identified then it is hopefully possible to either avoid them or at least reduce one's exposure. Relaxation techniques, such as breathing exercises and other complementary therapies (*see* Part Two of the book), are helpful both for prevention and treatment. Taking regular, daily exercise and allowing sufficient time for sleep have both been identified as important. Exercise helps to reduce stress and depression, both of which are common causes of headaches. Tiredness is frequently implicated in the generation of headaches and sometimes all that is needed is an adjustment to your daily routine and recognition of the importance of a good night's sleep.

Chapter 4

CLUSTER HEADACHES

(Alternative names: *Alarm clock headache, suicide headache, Horton's headache, histamine headache, ciliary neuralgia, petrosal neuralgia, hemicranial neuralgiformis chronica, erythroprosopalgia of Bing, migrainous neuralgia*)

What are cluster headaches?

Cluster headaches are a highly distinctive type of headache when compared to either tension headaches or migraines. Although their existence has been recognised medically for over a century, they remain commonly misdiagnosed and consequently sometimes inadequately managed and treated. This is despite the fact that the pain involved is widely acknowledged to be both excruciating and highly disabling for sufferers of the condition. Most of those affected describe the pain as the worst that they have ever experienced or could imagine experiencing while women commonly claim that it is far more severe than the pain of childbirth. Given these facts, it is fortunate that cluster headaches are classed as rare although estimates of how many people are affected vary considerably.

While cluster headaches can occur at any age, they usually arise initially in adults between 20 and 40 years old and they are not thought to affect children. The incidence in the UK may be anything between 56 to 279 people in every 100,000 and the condition is 4 to 5 times more likely to affect men. Overall, there may be between 34,000 and 150,000 sufferers of the condition in the whole of the UK.

Cluster headaches are so named because they most usually occur in bouts, arising frequently during a specific time period, termed *the cluster period*. This is followed by a length of time when the person is headache-free, termed *the remission period*. This typical pattern is sometimes given the title *episodic cluster headaches* and it is by far the most common manifestation of the disorder.

Within this overall pattern, other trends are normally present. Firstly, the headaches typically begin at the same time each day, commonly during the period of night-time sleep (hence, *alarm clock headache*). Very often, the person is awakened by the headache about an hour and a half after first falling asleep, during the phase of rapid eye movement (REM) sleep that is recognised by specialists. Individuals who experience night-time cluster headaches or who have a cluster headache on awakening may also be suffering from sleep apnea (when a person temporarily stops breathing) which tends to intensify cluster headaches. Many may not be aware that they have this condition and so do not seek any help for the problem. Secondly, the active cluster period is normally seasonal, occurring at the same time of year and often during the spring or autumn. A further characteristic is that the headaches are one-sided and during any particular cluster period, they rarely change sides.

Individual headaches usually occur rapidly, coming on within about 10 minutes, generally without prior warning. They typically last for anything between half an hour to 3 hours but most commonly, for 20 minutes to 90 minutes. Headaches may occur once every 2 days or far more frequently, up to 8 or more times each day.

The length of the cluster period varies considerably. Typically, it lasts for about 6 to 12 weeks but it may be shorter or longer than this. The remission phase is equally variable in length and in rare cases only one cluster period is ever experienced. Periods of remission may last for many years but, more usually, there is a cluster phase either annually or biannually. Even during the remission phase, some people occasionally experience minor bouts of 'break-through' headaches, perhaps lasting for just a few days.

In about 10% of all cases, bouts continue without remission and if this happens, the person is deemed to be suffering from *chronic cluster headaches*. A further extremely unusual form, which almost exclusively affects women, is called *chronic paraoxysmal hemicrania*. The headaches are of even greater severity, always occur on the same side of the head and are short-lived, lasting from between 5 minutes to 30 minutes. But they arise as multiple attacks of perhaps as many as 15 to 30 headaches per day and are highly disabling and debilitating for the person concerned.

Although a cluster headache most usually arises without prior warning, a few people report a preceding feeling of heaviness or a dull ache. In all instances, the pain is commonly described as being 'sharp', 'piercing', 'burning', 'stabbing' or 'needle-like' and it is centred around one eye and the temple on the same side. Sometimes the pain spreads more widely and it may extend into the neck and very rarely it is described as throbbing. The eye on the affected side frequently becomes inflamed, bloodshot and streams profusely. The eyelids often swell and they may droop (ptosis) and sometimes the pupil of the affected eye becomes contracted. The nose on that side often becomes congested and sweating of the face is commonly present.

The pain of a cluster headache has a severely disabling effect while it lasts and typically produces agitated behaviour. The person may repetitively pace in circles or up and down and even strike the body or head in an effort to provide a distraction.

Not surprisingly, in individuals who suffer from cluster headaches there is a significant risk of depression and even suicide and it is very important for those affected to receive effective treatment and help to cope with the condition. Anyone who suspects he (or she) may be affected by cluster headaches should certainly seek medical help from their GP (with probably an onward referral to a specialist headache clinic) and if their headaches are occurring at night, they can also ask about the possibility of sleep apnea making their headaches worse.

Causes

The precise cause of cluster headaches remains unknown but research has revealed some interesting clues. It has been established that a region of the brain called the hypothalamus is activated ipsilaterally (on one side) during an attack and this area has direct connections with both the trigeminal nerve and cranial parasympathetic nerves. Hence it is believed that a dysfunction within the hypothalamus starts off the chain of events that leads to the generation of cluster headaches. When this occurs, there is a release of neurotransmitters (naturally occurring biochemical substances involved in the transmission of electrical impulses), resulting in stimulation of the trigeminal nerve and parasympathetic nerve network, along with dilation of cranial blood vessels.

It has been discovered that hypoxaemia (a lowered level of oxygen in the blood), which naturally causes blood vessels to dilate, is associated with the causation of cluster headaches. The carotid body is a specialised area within the large carotid arteries through which the brain is supplied with blood and it is involved in monitoring the levels of oxygen and carbon dioxide. It is possible that this may be a further feedback mechanism that is involved in some way. The exact mechanism is highly complex but it is thought that the dysfunction in the hypothalamus causes the dilation of cranial blood vessels within the brain and that this is brought about by stimulation of the trigeminal nerve and the operation of reflexes in the parasympathetic nervous system. The result of this combined series of events is the generation of the one-sided pain and accompanying autonomic symptoms (brought about by the part of the nervous system not under conscious control) such as the watery eye and blocked nose characteristic of the condition.

The situation is further complicated by the fact that the hypothalamus is involved in the regulation of the internal 'body clock' in all higher mammals, including human beings. It is involved in the regulation not only of circadian (daily) rhythms but of circannual (yearly) ones as well. These regulatory mechanisms are responsive to both daily and seasonal changes in cycles of light and dark known as photoperiodic changes. A hormone called melatonin is known to be a key factor in their operation.

Melatonin is a naturally occurring biochemical substance that is secreted by the pineal gland (a small, highly specialised mass of nerve tissue located near the centre of the brain). This hormone is involved in the regulation of circadian rhythms in all higher mammals. More specifically, it is involved in bringing about the changes in activity, behaviour and physiology that occur during any 24-hour period, such as the determination of phases of sleep and wakefulness. In normal circumstances, melatonin is released at high levels during the hours of darkness but its secretion is low and suppressed during the day. The levels of the hormone vary not only daily but also on a seasonal basis, connected with changes in the amount of daylight. In mammals, it is thought that melatonin has a role in determining circannual rhythms such as the breeding season and hibernation.

Critically with regard to cluster headaches, it has been discovered that altered levels of the hormone are found in sufferers of the condition and it is likely that other naturally occurring biochemical substances involved in regulation are similarly affected.

One other interesting link is that among affected men, lowered plasma levels of testosterone are found both throughout a cluster period and during an attack. Taken together, these findings have opened up the possibility of potentially helpful treatments and preventatives in the management of the condition, such as melatonin replacement therapy and light therapy.

Finally, recent studies have revealed that genetic factors are also implicated and the gene involved is designated HCRTR2. The gene shows an autosomal dominant pattern of inheritance and its presence is connected with an increased risk of cluster headaches. About 1 in 20 sufferers have a close family member who is similarly afflicted. In general, a close relative of someone affected is at a higher risk of cluster headaches than a person without such a connection.

In the majority of cases, individual headaches usually arise without warning. However, certain *triggers* have been identified as being important in some people and as they are potential risk factors for all sufferers of the condition, it is useful to highlight them here. In general, triggers are only significant within the duration of the cluster period and do not have the same influence at other times.

Cluster headache triggers

ALCOHOL is of particular importance and it is the most commonly reported trigger of cluster headaches. The best advice is to avoid alcoholic drinks altogether during the cluster period and to proceed cautiously outside this time, especially near to the beginning or end of the headache period.

SUBSTANCES WITH A PUNGENT SMELL such as perfumes, strongly scented air fresheners, paints, petrol and similar industrial chemicals and solvents may also act as triggers. It is particularly important to avoid inhaling any volatile substance known to cause dilation of blood vessels such as nitro-glycerine, as this is likely to provoke an attack.

EXCESSIVE HEAT can be a trigger, extending even to taking a hot bath or becoming warm with exercise.

STRENUOUS PHYSICAL ACTIVITY is a trigger in some people and it may be advisable to take only gentle to moderate exercise during the cluster period.

SMOKING – a majority of those affected by cluster headaches are, or have previously been, smokers. Although there is no supporting evidence to suggest that giving up smoking reduces the occurrence of headaches, it is undoubtedly the case that this will improve general health and lessen the risk of other serious illnesses.

See also **A Summary of the Environmental and Lifestyle Causes of Headaches** on page 53.

Treatment

Treatment for cluster headaches operates on two fronts: firstly, to abort or relieve a headache that has started; and secondly, to prevent the headaches from occurring. In practice, there is a considerable degree of overlap between these two approaches, and the use of some drugs is restricted to one or other of the particular forms of cluster headaches. With regard to treatment, it is the case that the ordinary, pain-relieving medications in common use are entirely ineffective. The prescription-only drugs that are used for the prevention and treatment of cluster headaches are not analgesics but work in an entirely different way.

Whatever medication you are given for your headache, it is very important that you:

- Read all the instructions that come with the packaging and follow the directions given by your doctor.
- Be aware of any side effects or cautions (some medications, for example, can make you feel very drowsy). If you are aware of any possible serious side effects, you will know to see a doctor straightaway if they do occur.
- Tell your doctor about any other medication you may be taking because some headache medicines can react badly with other medicines.

The drug that is most widely prescribed is called sumatriptan and it is also used to treat migraine. Pharmacologically, it belongs to the triptans group and these act upon a naturally occurring biochemical substance called 5-hydroxytryptamine (5-HT) or serotonin. Serotonin is a derivative of an amino acid (protein) called tryptophan and it functions as a neurotransmitter but is also involved in the dilation and contraction of blood vessels. It is found in the brain and nervous system and also in some other areas of the body, including the gut. As described above, both the nervous and circulatory systems are involved in the generation of cluster headaches. It is believed that alterations in the level of 5-HT are directly implicated, particularly in relation to dilation of cranial blood vessels. The mode of action of sumatriptan is mainly as a 5-HT1 receptor agonist. This means that it has an attraction or affinity for 5-HT receptors, competing for their use and thereby reducing the number available to 5-HT, thus reducing its physiological effects.

Sumatriptan is not able to cross the blood-brain-barrier (BBB) which is believed to be both a physiological and anatomical feature of certain blood capillaries in the brain. It operates to exclude, slow down and generally regulate the inward and outward flow of various compounds, biochemical substances and foreign bodies between the blood circulation and the brain. It is therefore thought that sumatriptan acts within the blood vessels of the meninges (the connective tissue membranes that surround the brain and spinal cord). The drug is classed as a first generation triptan and it has a low bioavailability of 14%, compared to that of more recently developed, second-generation triptans, and its period of physiological activity is relatively short. However, it is quick-acting.

Sumatriptan can be taken orally but it is usually self-administered in the form of a subcutaneous injection, commonly employing an 'auto-injector' device containing a preloaded syringe that delivers the correct dose. Use of the drug is most effective if administered as soon as the headache starts. In most cases, the drug becomes active within 5 to 10 minutes. The adult dose is 6 mg per headache, with a maximum permissible daily dose of 12 mg – hence 2 injections in any 24-hour period – and there must be an interval of at least an hour between the injections.

Side effects may be experienced but generally these are mild. They include a dry mouth, dizziness, nausea and a sense of weariness. A small number of people may experience other symptoms such as flushing and a feeling of warmth, sensations of tightness or tingling and a feeling of pressure in the limbs and occasionally across the chest. Any side effects should be reported and discussed with the doctor prescribing the medication. Sumatriptan is contraindicated in some patients, including those who have suffered or are at risk of stroke, heart problems or peripheral circulatory disorders.

Ergotamine is another drug that may be used in treatment and it is administered either orally or as a rectal suppository. The dose must be strictly controlled both on a daily and weekly basis to avoid potentially harmful side effects and the drug can only be taken for short, intermittent periods. Ergotamine works by causing temporary contraction of blood vessels and so it is unsuitable for patients suffering from any form of circulatory disorder. Dihydroergotamine is an injectable form and again, this has to be used cautiously. When injected, there is a greater risk of side effects such as nausea.

Oxygen is a non-drug therapy that is effective in about three quarters of all patients although it may not abort every individual headache. Portable cylinders can be supplied for home use and the patient simply breathes the pure oxygen through a face mask at the onset of a headache.

Prevention

Preventative or prophylactic preparations are also prescribed for use during a cluster period in the episodic form of the condition. Ergotamine is used in this way and it is commonly taken at bedtime before the person goes to sleep, or an hour or two before the expected time of onset of a headache.

Verapamil, lithium and divalproex are a further three medications prescribed in tablet form for oral administration. They may all be used in the prevention of episodic cluster headache or, as a continual treatment for the chronic form of the condition. Patients prescribed verapamil require close monitoring of the heart by means of electroencephalogram (ECG) recordings, especially if the dosage is being increased. If lithium is being taken, the condition of blood vessels must be monitored, as there is a risk of unwanted side effects.

Methysergide is an effective preventative drug but it is generally only prescribed on a last-chance basis when other preparations have failed. It can only be used for a maximum period of six months and so it is of limited value for chronic cluster headaches.

Prednisone is often effective in bringing a cluster period to an end. It is generally used for a limited period of around 2 to 4 weeks, the dose being gradually reduced but it is not prescribed for the chronic form of the condition. Other corticosteroid preparations are sometimes prescribed for short-term use at the start of a cluster period but cannot be used longer term due to the risk of adverse steroid side effects. A corticosteroid preparation may be used alongside another drug, such as verapamil, at the start of treatment, but then it is gradually phased out as the main medication builds up and begins to take effect.

Indomethacin is a drug particularly used to treat chronic paroxysmal hemicrania (CPH) but it is not prescribed either for treatment or prevention of other forms of cluster headache.

Chapter 5

MIGRAINE HEADACHES

What is a migraine headache?

A migraine is a distinctive form of recurrent, severe headache that often occurs as 'attacks' or episodes of pain but without any apparent seasonal pattern or periodicity. The pain is often (but not exclusively) confined to one side of the head and is characteristically accompanied by certain other symptoms and manifestations. About 20% of all the headaches experienced in the UK at any particular time are migraines.

Approximately 15% (some 6 million people) of the population in the UK are sufferers and about 66% of these are female. Children can be affected (see **Headaches in Children** on page 51) but the onset of migraines usually coincides with puberty. Boys tend to be affected at a younger age while among girls the first attack often occurs around the same time as the onset of menstrual periods. In general, migraines most commonly affect younger adults aged between their mid-teens and early 40s.

The number of attacks varies greatly but on average, a sufferer experiences about 15 migraines in every year. Some people may go for years without an attack and in others, individual migraines only occur occasionally. But in those severely affected, headaches can occur as frequently as several times a week and have a serious and disabling effect upon their enjoyment and quality of life.

The duration of the pain of a single migraine can be anything from 4 hours to 2 or 3 days and, quite often, the person feels tired and 'washed out' for a day or so afterwards. Between attacks there are no symptoms but it is possible for a migraine sufferer to experience an ordinary tension headache at other times.

Two main types of migraine are recognised: *migraine without aura* or *common migraine* and *migraine with aura* or *classical migraine*. Also, there are some atypical, unusual forms and in some cases, these may be linked to other (genetic) factors.

Migraine without aura

Migraine without aura is the type most commonly experienced by about 90% of all those affected by migraine. The symptoms are:

- A moderate to severe headache develops, usually on one side although a feeling of pressure may be felt throughout the head and sometimes pain extends down into the neck. The headache is typically dull to begin with but it increases in severity over a period of 2 to 12 hours, when it reaches a peak. However, it may also be severe from the start. The pain is described as intense, severe, throbbing or pulsating and moving the head usually makes it worse. The pain subsides gradually, over a variable period of time.

And one or more of the following is commonly experienced:

- Nausea, vomiting.
- Photophobia – an increased sensitivity and intolerance of light, often making it necessary to lie down in a darkened room.

- An increased sensitivity and intolerance of sound, even of moderate levels of everyday noise.
- An increased sensitivity and intolerance of odours, such as those from foodstuffs, drinks, perfume, etc.
- There may also be blurring of vision, sweating, shivering, loss of concentration, sense of slight disorientation, dizziness, abdominal pain, diarrhoea, increased urination, blocked nose, tender scalp and feelings of hunger.

Migraine with aura

In this more rare form of the condition, the headache and other symptoms are the same as those described above but they are preceded by certain neurological disturbances known as *aura*. Usually, people suffering from migraine with aura are able to tell when an attack is imminent. They may feel excited or euphoric, unaccustomedly hungry or thirsty or have cravings for certain foods or feel irritable and depressed. None of these may be present but just an uncanny 'sixth sense' that a migraine is about to occur.

The aura itself usually lasts from just a few minutes to up to an hour but in some cases, for a great deal longer than this. It is common for the headache to arise within an hour of the disappearance of the aura. However, if the aura is long lasting then it may continue for the duration of the pain or at least persist for part of the headache period.

The most common type of aura is some form of visual disturbance including seeing zigzag patterns, flashing lights or a rippling effect or even a temporary partial loss of sight. Sometimes objects within view appear to be shaking or distorted. The second most frequently reported manifestation is a spreading sense of numbness or 'pins-and-needles'. The sensation often travels from a hand on one side, up the arm and to the neck and face where the nose and mouth may be affected. The numbness may also be felt in a lower limb or limbs. In severe cases, there can be a loss or partial loss of speech, confusion, fainting and degrees of temporary paralysis. When experienced for the first time, these very frightening symptoms can be mistaken for a stroke.

People affected by this form of migraine may sometimes experience the aura without the development of a headache. Also, it is common for sufferers to have migraine without aura on some occasions.

Combining the two forms, doctors recognise five stages of migraine although not every stage is present in all cases.

1. The *prodromal* or *premonition stage* – the early warning period when signs of, or a sense of, an impending attack are present.
2. The *aura stage*.
3. The *headache stage*.
4. The *resolution stage* describes the period when symptoms gradually subside. In some people, vomiting brings about an immediate cessation of the headache. Others wake up pain free after a period of sleep.
5. The *postdromal* or *recovery stage* refers to the period when all symptoms have disappeared. The person may feel weak, exhausted and dispirited for up to 24 hours and sometimes for even longer than this.

Causes

The exact causes of migraine are not fully understood but it is thought that some of the same mechanisms that are implicated in cluster headaches are also at work in migraine. The principle factors appear to be the trigemino-vascular system (the trigeminal nerve and peripheral blood vessels in the brain) and the neurotransmitter 5-HT or serotonin. Receptors in the nerve and blood vessels are serotonergic (sensitive to serotonin) and the level of this is known to decrease at the start of a migraine headache. Activation of the trigemino-vascular system, which takes place during a migraine, is involved in causing the contraction and expansion of blood vessels and the generation of pain. The reasons why some people are susceptible while others are not have yet to be explained. It is possible that sufferers may have a more highly sensitive pain centre within the brain but it is likely that several factors act in combination to determine whether an individual is affected or not. It is now believed that there is a genetic predisposition for migraine headaches with aura and this is supported by the fact that about 80% of migraine sufferers have another family member who is also affected. It is hoped that this finding will in time lead to a target for therapies.

Migraine attack triggers

A trigger is any activity, event or substance that provokes a migraine attack. Almost anything can act as a trigger but something to which one individual is sensitive may not cause an attack in someone else. Confusingly, even when a person is able to identify a trigger, it may not cause an attack on every single occasion. Some sufferers are able to discover one or more triggers while others cannot identify a single factor with any degree of certainty. The majority of attacks appear to occur without any obvious trigger although it may be that this is due, at least some of the time, to a failure of identification rather than true absence. It may also be the case that one or more triggers combine, such as stress or tiredness coupled with a missed meal.

The list of known, identified, common triggers includes:

- Foods, including chocolate, dairy products (especially cheese and particularly mature or strong-flavoured varieties), smoked fish, red wine and other alcoholic drinks,

pickled and fermented foods, processed foods and meats, coffee, foods containing monosodium glutamate or artificial sweeteners, citrus fruits, vegetables, yeast products, highly coloured oriental foods, fried foods, frozen pizzas.
- Hypoglycaemia due to irregular or missed meals and insufficient food intake.
- Stress and emotional factors such as anger.
- Relaxation at the end of a period of stress.
- Tiredness or disruption of sleep pattern including excess sleep.
- Eye-strain.
- Poor posture, neck and back strain.
- Cigarette smoke.
- Teeth grinding during sleep.
- Changes in weather.
- Bright or flashing lights.
- Loud or sudden noises.
- Certain odours including perfumes, petrol and paint.
- Physical exertion or too little exercise.
- Travelling or long journeys.
- Other drug preparations.
- In women, hormonal changes. The levels of female hormones fluctuate naturally during the menstrual cycle and evidence proves that women are susceptible to migraine attack at the onset of a period, when oestrogen is at its lowest level. Also, migraines often disappear during pregnancy. The combined oral contraceptive pill and HRT are not advised for women suffering from migraine with aura. Those with severe migraine may be at higher risk of stroke if they take preparations containing oestrogen. It is sensible for all female sufferers to seek medical advice about the advisability of taking hormonal preparations and to inform their doctor if any changes are noticed while taking medication.

Treatment

Analgesic (pain-relieving) medication can often be effective in alleviating migraine, especially if the attack is a mild one. It works best if taken as soon as symptoms appear but is much less likely to be effective if delayed until the pain has increased in severity. The fact that analgesics are less effective at the peak of an attack is well established. This is partly because there is less absorption through the stomach wall at this time, particularly if there is nausea or vomiting. If tablets have been swallowed, they may just lie in the stomach or even be vomited up, rather than being absorbed. For this reason, it may be helpful to choose soluble or effervescent preparations that are more readily absorbed into the blood circulation. Nasal sprays, anal or vaginal suppositories and injections are other potential alternative methods of drug delivery.

Over-the-counter preparations such as paracetamol, ibuprofen and aspirin (the latter not recommended for children) can be tried. Stronger painkillers, including diclofenac, tolfenamic acid and naproxen are available only on prescription. Antisickness (antiemetic) medicines can be taken along with analgesics and once again, these are most effective if taken at the start of an attack. Some over-the-counter preparations especially formulated for migraine such as *Migraleve*, *Paramax* and *Migramax* combine analgesics (paracetamol and codeine) with antiemetic drugs. However the ratios of active ingredients in these combinations may not be optimal for every individual and it can be more helpful to take antiemetics, such as metoclopramide or domperidone, separately so that doses can be adjusted to suit. These are prescription medications and they can, once again, be delivered by alternative means such as suppositories, if required.

Other medication used in treatment comprises drugs known as triptans. Members of this family are 5-HT1 receptor agonists that work by correcting the imbalances in serotonin levels that arise during a migraine attack (see also page 32). Various drugs are available including sumatriptan (the mainstay of treatment), fovatriptan, rizatriptan, zolmitriptan, eletriptan, almotriptan and naratriptan. Only four of these are licensed for use in the UK: sumatriptan (available as *Imigran* and *Imitrex*); naratriptan (*Amerge* and *Naramig*); rizatriptan (*Maxalt*) and zolmitriptan (*Zomig*). It may be necessary for several of these to be tried before discovering the one that is most suitable. All of them can produce side effects, including nausea, vomiting, stiffness or pressure in the neck, chest and in other parts of the body. The preparations are not suitable for elderly people aged over 65 or anyone with existing heart or circulatory disease, high blood pressure or at risk of stroke.

If migraines are very severe and particularly if other drugs have proved ineffective, other medication may be prescribed. Often these are highly potent, one example being ergotamine tartrate, but this is unsuitable for anyone with heart, circulatory or kidney problems or for women who are pregnant or breastfeeding.

Whatever the medication being taken, most sufferers find it helpful to rest or lie down in a quiet, darkened room while an attack is being experienced. Placing an ice pack or cold flannel on the head may provide some relief.

Prevention

If triggers have been identified then avoidance of these as far as possible is one obvious helpful measure that can be employed. However, as with other types of headache, prevention of migraine attacks can be problematic. Prophylactic medication can be prescribed but generally, it lessens frequency and severity rather than aborting attacks altogether. The drugs that are prescribed are taken on a daily basis, irrespective of anything that is used during an actual attack. They include beta-blockers such as propanolol (*Inderal A*, but not suitable for those with asthma), antidepressants such as amitryptyline, antihistamines such as pizotifen which is usually taken at night as it can cause drowsiness, anticonvulsants such as topiramate and sodium valproate (*Epilin*, but not licensed for migraine treatment). All these are potent preparations with a range of potential side effects and contraindications. They can only be prescribed after careful medical evaluation and consultation.

Other preventative measures that are said to be helpful for some people include wearing tinted glasses, wearing dental splints at night to prevent teeth grinding (if applicable), physiotherapy and certain complementary therapies, e.g. the herb, Feverfew, has been found to be effective for some sufferers when taken on a daily basis, but medical advice should be obtained before taking this herb. It is also important to try and sit correctly, maintain a good posture and to take regular exercise.

Depression is more common among those affected by migraine and conversely, sufferers with depression are at greater risk of having migraine attacks. Research is currently underway to try and determine if successful treatment for depression is, in itself, a method of prevention.

Rare forms of migraine

Opthalmoplegic or *ocular migraine* is characterised by lateral pain, usually centred around one eye, with accompanying double vision or other vision disturbance. Nausea and vomiting are commonly present. *Hemiplegic migraine* produces symptoms that are sometimes confused with a stroke but they are generally entirely reversible. There is double vision or other vision disturbance, temporary blindness and degrees of deafness, short-lived, one-sided paralysis and facial numbness causing speech and swallowing difficulties. All these symptoms may be present to a greater or lesser extent and effects may persist for several days before wearing off entirely. *Basilar artery migraine* can rarely arise during an attack and it arises when the basilar artery, which supplies blood to the base of the brain, enters into spasm. Symptoms include double vision, giddiness, fainting and loss of consciousness and they are caused by a lowered oxygen supply to the brain. For *abdominal migraine, see* **Headaches in Children** on page 51.

Migraine and epilepsy

Some people suffer from both migraine and epilepsy (a brain disorder triggered by an abnormal neural discharge resulting in seizures). Although these are two quite distinct conditions, they share some of the same symptoms, e.g. visual disturbances, and the same triggers, e.g. stress, lack of sleep and hormonal fluctuation. It is important if you suffer from migraines as well as seizures that you inform your doctor. Anticonvulsant medication used to treat epilepsy has also been used with some success to treat people who have migraine attacks, but some drugs may be appropriate for one condition and have detrimental effects on the other. If you do suffer from both migraines and epilepsy, treatment can sometimes collectively address both conditions.

Chapter 6

CHRONIC DAILY HEADACHES (CDH)

What are chronic daily headaches?

Chronic daily headaches can comprise one or more of the three main types and it is estimated that 3% to 4% of people in the UK are affected. The condition can arise in people of any age, from young children to elderly persons, and it is common for sufferers to experience some degree of neck stiffness and muscle contraction in addition to pain. Almost half of those who consult their GP about headaches are suffering from this form of disorder. They are most likely to fall within the age range of 30 to 40 years and to have been affected by tension headaches or migraines for some considerable time.

Causes

The most common cause of CDH is overuse of analgesic drugs, most frequently those formulations that can be bought over-the-counter in pharmacies and supermarkets. This has led to CDH being afforded certain other titles including *analgesic rebound*, *medication misuse* or *medication overuse headaches*. It is estimated that about a fifth of sufferers of CDH fall into the medication overuse category and among this group, women outnumber men by 5 to 1.

In many cases, the medication was taken in the first instance to relieve the pain of headaches and it has now been established that use of analgesics for only a few days each week can cause the problem. But in many cases, sufferers have taken considerably more analgesics than this and have also used more than one type and typically, those affected have a long-standing medical history of tension headaches or migraine.

All analgesics are implicated in causing the problem but it is thought that compound preparations, such as those combining aspirin and paracetamol, pose a greater risk. It has also been established that small doses (possibly less than the recommended daily allowance) taken every day are more likely to cause analgesic rebound headaches than larger doses that are only taken occasionally. In addition to painkillers, ergotamine and drugs of the triptans group, often prescribed for cluster headaches and migraines are also implicated, as is caffeine.

CDH is often at its most severe upon first waking up in the morning and the pain is also made worse with exertion and exercise. Depression and sleep disturbance are commonplace and CDH can have a profound effect upon a sufferer's quality of life and ability to function normally.

A diagnosis requires taking details of the patient's medical history and subjecting this record to thorough analysis. Before CDH can be laid at the door of analgesic rebound, other potential causes and medical problems must be explored and eliminated.

Treatment

Appropriate treatment depends upon the cause being correctly identified and a different approach may be needed if analgesics are being taken for other forms of pain such as arthritic or rheumatic problems. Some patients may have a musculo-skeletal problem or psychological and emotional problems that must also be addressed. If analgesic misuse is found to be at the root of the problem, treatment consists of gradual withdrawal of the medication combined with counselling and patient education. The majority of patients respond well to treatment and although they may not become completely free of headaches altogether, there is usually a considerable reduction in frequency. Other prescription drugs, usually antidepressant or anti-epileptic medication, may be helpful for some patients. Preparations include prednisolone, tricyclic antidepressants such as nor-triptylline and anitryptiline, anti-epileptics, e.g. sodium valproate, topiramate and garbapentin, and beta-blockers, such as propanolol. These are all potent drugs and careful evaluation of each person's needs is required before they can be prescribed. They may not be suitable for all sufferers of CDH and certain pre-existing medical conditions and disorders may rule out their use in some cases.

Chapter 7

KEEPING A HEADACHE DIARY

If headaches are occurring on a regular basis and at a level that is interfering with a person's ability to lead a normal life, it might be useful to record the attacks by keeping a headache diary. This can be a useful aid both for the sufferer and his (or her) doctor in discovering whether there is any discernible pattern or common factors in the occurrence of the headaches. The diary may be of use both before and after diagnosis as an aid to the longer-term management of the condition. A range of factors should be noted on a daily basis for a period of about six months, with the occurrence of each headache recorded, including the time the pain begins, its intensity, any medication taken and the duration of the attack. Factors that should be noted include:

- Time of waking.
- Duration or pattern of sleep.
- Meals and foods – meal times and foods consumed, including drinks and alcohol.
- Weather.
- Mood and wellbeing.
- In women, the time and duration of periods.

- Bowel movements.
- Travel and journeys.
- Environment – exposure to noise, fumes, pollutants, sunlight.
- Season.
- Stressful events.
- Medication taken including that for conditions other than headaches.
- Time of going to sleep and activity before sleep.
- Any other factors that may be relevant.

While it is by no means certain that a pattern will emerge, keeping a headache diary is, in itself, a positive, self-help step that can be taken. It helps the person to feel more in control and to engender a positive mental attitude.

Chapter 8

HEADACHES IN CHILDREN

Children suffer from the same type of headaches as adults and for similar reasons. It used to be thought that newborn babies and very young infants did not suffer pain in the same way as older children but it is now realised that the difficulty lay in measuring pain in this age group. Even so, it is difficult to ascertain whether a baby is suffering from a headache or experiencing it in the same way as an older child or adult. But it is possible that even a newborn baby could be affected and there is now a greater degree of understanding of the effects of a traumatic delivery on generating skeletal problems and pain, which might include headache.

Young children have difficulty in accurately pinpointing the source of pain and of course a child who is ill and feverish may also be crying and distressed. A headache is very likely to be present in these circumstances. Children are most likely to be affected by tension headaches or migraines, with cluster headaches being a rare occurrence. They are also far more susceptible than adults to headaches caused by hypoglycaemia (low blood sugar) or dehydration (insufficient fluid intake), simply because of their smaller body size. It is essential to ensure that children eat regularly and that they have a good, healthy diet and drink plenty of fluids, preferably plain water, especially during hot weather. Infants are unable to regulate their body temperature efficiently and dehydration is a particular risk in young children. Many of the sweet, fizzy drinks that children enjoy are diuretic to a certain extent due to the high sugar and/or caffeine content. While children are very young, it is sensible to avoid these drinks altogether and to encourage older ones to drink water on a regular basis, to avoid dehydration.

Children most commonly suffer from tension headaches caused by such factors as lack of sleep, stress, over-excitement, foods, additives or artificial colouring in food and drinks, and environmental substances such as fumes or smoke. In rare cases, tension headaches can occur on a regular basis and become chronic and this obviously requires careful treatment. In most cases, over-the-counter preparations especially formulated for children are effective in dealing with pain. If there are other factors involved, some adjustments to the child's routine may be needed to lessen the chance of recurrence.

A proportion of children afflicted by headaches are diagnosed as suffering from migraine. Often there is genetic basis for the condition with other family members similarly affected. Some young children suffer from an unusual form called *abdominal migraine* in which pain is felt in the abdomen rather than the head. There may be accompanying nausea and vomiting and aura may be present but usually, headache pain is either mild or absent. Children with this form of the condition commonly develop a typical migraine pattern once they become adolescents.

Prescription medications may be needed for treatment and prevention and these are generally the same as those used for adults.

Chapter 9

A SUMMARY OF THE ENVIRONMENTAL AND LIFESTYLE CAUSES OF HEADACHES

Many of the factors included in this section have already been described in earlier chapters but it is useful to summarise them since they fall, at least to a certain extent, within an individual's control and hence can potentially either be avoided or their effects mitigated.

Alcohol

Alcohol, especially if consumed to excess and so producing the classic symptoms of a 'hangover', is a common and entirely avoidable cause of pounding, painful headaches. Alcohol is implicated as a cause of many other serious medical conditions and disorders in addition to headaches. The best advice is to follow the current health guidelines and to limit consumption so as not to exceed 21 units each week for men and 14 for women. The daily limit should be around 2 to 3 units for men and 1 to 2 for women (approximately equating to a smallish glass of wine). It is best to drink alcohol with a meal and to match each alcoholic drink with a similar volume of water. Binge drinking should always be avoided. For most people, drinking at this modest level should not cause headaches. But many people of Chinese ethnic origin are unable to metabolise alcohol due to a physiological lack of a particular enzyme and have an unpleasant reaction, even to a small amount. Likewise, if alcohol is a known trigger for your headaches then it may be sensible to avoid it altogether.

Food and drink

Certain other drinks and foods are a well-known cause of headaches in people who are sensitive to the particular substance involved. Almost any substance can be implicated but well-recognised ones include chocolate, cheese, caffeine (coffee, tea, certain carbonated drinks, dark chocolate), food dyes and other additives, sweeteners and preservatives.

Hypoglycaemia and dehydration

Low blood-sugar levels and mild dehydration are common headache causes that are likely to be experienced by many people at some stage in life. It is important to eat regular meals containing complex carbohydrates (high fibre, starchy foods) as these promote a slow release of glucose into the bloodstream and a steady supply of energy. Highly refined, sweet foods are more likely to produce peaking of blood sugar and favour the development of obesity and diabetes.

Our modern busy lifestyles favour the occurrence of slight dehydration with people sometimes forgetting to drink, either because of lack of opportunity or failure to listen to the promptings of thirst. Often, by the end of the working day, the result of this is a slight, nagging headache. It is sensible to keep a glass or bottle of water to hand and to take frequent sips in order to avoid this problem and it is particularly important to do this when conditions are hot and dry.

Stress and anxiety

Stress and anxiety are hard to avoid altogether and are recognised as a frequent cause of headaches. People can be unaware that they are experiencing undue levels of stress and fail to do anything to address the problem. There are many simple ways to lessen the effects, from going for a walk to practising relaxation to ensuring that you allow enough time for restful sleep (see appropriate complementary therapies in the second part of the book). If prolonged, high levels of stress are damaging to health and wellbeing and can be a cause of many other types of illness, some of them severe such as heart disease and mental disorders.

In some instances it is not the stress that causes the migraine but the relaxation that follows a period of stress hence the name *letdown migraine* or *letdown headache* which is usually applied to this sort of migraine headache.

Sleep disorders

Sleep disorders, especially insomnia and disruption of the normal pattern of sleep, frequently accompany stress, anxiety, depression and mental illness and can also be a feature of other conditions such as the menopause. Disturbance of sleep is a well-known cause of headaches and one that most people experience occasionally. If the disruption continues for any length of time, headaches may arise quite frequently and medical advice should be sought. Short-term use of sleeping pills may be helpful to try and overcome the problem.

Exercise

Exercise can be a cause and, in this context, it is not only hard, physical effort that is implicated but also exertion associated with everyday life. Coughing, sneezing, straining to open the bowels, sexual activity and lifting heavy weights can all cause headaches in some people. If the problem is persistent or occurs suddenly without happening previously then medical advice should be sought. Constipation can usually be relieved by a change of diet or short-term use of laxatives. Care should always be taken to lift heavy weights correctly, not only to avoid headaches but also to avoid damaging the back.

Environmental pollution

Environmental pollution, whether the source is excess noise, light or fumes, is a recognised cause of headaches. In our modern, industrial world pollution of this nature is an ever-increasing problem and one that is hard to avoid altogether. However, avoidance, especially in the home is probably the best way for a susceptible person to try and lessen the triggering of headaches.

Carbon monoxide poisoning

Carbon monoxide poisoning is a rare cause of headaches but, unfortunately, some cases occur each year in the UK and some of these are fatal. The danger lies in the fact that carbon monoxide is a colourless and odourless gas and is highly poisonous when inhaled. It is present in vehicle exhaust emissions and in coal gas and many cases of accidental poisoning arise due to faulty working of domestic gas heating boilers and appliances. Carbon monoxide (CO) enters the blood stream from the lungs and has a high affinity for the oxygen carrying molecule, haemoglobin. It readily binds to haemoglobin to form bright-red carboxyhaemoglobin and if the process continues, eventually there is no free haemoglobin left to collect oxygen and transport it to all the body's organs and tissues. The symptoms of poisoning include headache, often severe, flushing (due to carboxyhaemoglobin in the blood), nausea, giddiness, a rise in respiratory and heartbeat rate and eventual coma, respiratory failure and death. It is not uncommon for the early symptoms to be mistaken for the onset of flu and it is especially dangerous if poisoning occurs at night while people are asleep as they may simply succumb without awakening. It is essential for all household gas appliances to be serviced on an annual basis and there should be adequate ventilation at all times. Anyone who suspects carbon monoxide poisoning should immediately get those affected outside into the fresh air, before summoning emergency medical help.

Altitude sickness

Altitude sickness (also known as *mountain sickness*) is usually a recreational cause of headache. It affects people (especially mountaineers) who are exposed to a high altitude to which the body is unaccustomed, usually because they have arrived at a height above 3,000 metres without allowing the body sufficient time to adjust to the lower oxygen levels and higher atmospheric pressures that are found at high altitude. The physiological response in these circumstances is deep and rapid breathing (hyperventilation) in an attempt to obtain more oxygen. Symptoms include a severe headache, nausea, exhaustion, rapid deep breathing and anxiety. Many people suffer these unpleasant effects for up to 48 hours before they subside as the body gradually adjusts.

There is also a risk of the more serious and potentially fatal condition of pulmonary oedema in which fluid collects in the lungs. In this instance, the person must be evacuated immediately to a lower altitude and will require treatment in hospital.

Experienced mountaineers often try to acclimatise by spending a day or two at one level before proceeding up to the next level but even this is not always sufficient. It is often difficult to predict whether an individual will be affected. Someone who falls victim on one mountaineering expedition can remain unaffected on the next. Usually, the symptoms are relatively mild but if severe and disabling, there is no alternative but to descend to a lower level.

Most organised mountaineering expeditions have one or more people in the group who are trained to recognise the signs and know when it is necessary to act. For the individual planning a visit to a high altitude destination, the best advice is to take time to acclimatise, drink plenty of water, suck glucose sweets and avoid consuming alcohol. If affected by altitude sickness, take painkillers, drink lots of water, try to eat a little and rest until the symptoms subside.

Caisson disease

Caisson disease or *compressed air illness* (commonly called *the bends*) is a potential cause of headaches and other serious symptoms in those who undertake deep water diving or who fly high performance (military) aircraft. The symptoms include pains in the joints (the bends), severe headache and dizziness (*decompression sickness*), chest pain, breathing difficulties, unconsciousness and, if not treated, paralysis and death. Treatment involves admittance to a decompression chamber and emergency medical aid, until the person's body has readjusted to normal surface pressures. The cause of the illness is the formation of nitrogen bubbles in the blood, which then accumulate in different parts of the body. The nitrogen bubbles hinder normal circulation of the blood in supplying the tissues with nutrients and oxygen. Treatment in a decompression chamber forces the nitrogen bubbles to redissolve in the blood.

Avoidance of the illness can only be achieved by a slow return to the surface, from the high pressure at depth to the lower pressure nearer to the surface, spending a certain amount of time at each level. Anyone who dives either occupationally or recreationally is required to undergo strict training so that the hazards are clearly understood and they must always dive with a partner. Commercial diving operations should always include provision for emergency treatment by appropriately trained medical staff, with a decompression chamber always available for use.

Chapter 10

EFFECTS OF HEADACHES AND MIGRAINES ON EVERYDAY LIFE

The experience of pain

Any form of pain that is anything other than mild has some effect upon the quality of life of the person affected for the duration of its presence. If the pain occurs as a short-lived and isolated experience then the effects are less likely to be significant even if, at the time, the pain is quite severe. People vary widely in their individual responses and perception of pain with some undoubtedly coping better than others. But this may well be because some people experience pain more acutely – they have a greater sensitivity to pain or a so-called lower 'pain threshold'.

The experience of pain continues to be something that is not always well understood and throws up many challenges for researchers and members of the medical profession. It is only comparatively recently that 'pain clinics' have become a feature of medical care but often these are geared towards providing help for people with cancer. It may not be easy for everyone with pain to access the specialist services provided by a pain clinic. The fact that the significance of pain is now more widely recognised is obviously welcome as it is not too long ago that anyone suffering from pain that was not connected with a life-threatening condition was expected to grit their teeth and deal with it, with very little in the way of professional help. Fortunately, the generally accepted view now is that pain other than that connected with giving the body a warning does not serve any useful purpose and can be highly debilitating, not only for the individuals concerned but also for wider society. This is because there are unseen 'costs' with regard to pain – not only the cost of medical treatment but effects upon relationships and economic activity.

Headache pain

So how do headaches and migraines fit into the overall picture of pain? As has been seen, headache pain not only varies in severity with regard to type but also with each attack and, coupled with this, individual people may themselves experience it differently one from another. It is undoubtedly true that, at its worst, headache pain is very severe and exerts a profound effect upon a sufferer's life and it has to be taken seriously. An afflicted person can often do no more than lie down and rest in a darkened room while the pain lasts. He (or she) may not be able to eat, sleep or even drink anything for very many hours and they should not attempt to drive or operate machinery. Hence the person may face, in the first instance, the problem of getting to a suitable place for recovery. Important work or social activities, engagements and events have to be curtailed and the person can do no more than focus entirely upon dealing with the pain. Significant life events can be seriously affected, including sitting exams and exam attainment, job interviews and career prospects, travel, family celebrations, such as weddings, fitness to undergo planned medical or dental procedures – even sitting with a loved one who is dying. Headaches do not strike at times which are convenient and due to the connection with stress, the opposite situation is more likely to arise.

Even if headaches are rarely experienced, these effects should not be underestimated but often, as has been seen, the attacks are repeated over and over again and the problem becomes a long-term one. If this is the case then all the adverse effects upon everyday life greatly increase in magnitude. A further factor may arise in that even while headache-free, a person may live in dread of the next attack and so their enjoyment of life is constantly affected.

In the worst cases, activities, events and opportunities may be refused or postponed from fear of an attack occurring. While this represents one end of an extreme, it is not unheard of. There is a risk of profound psychological disorders, including depression and suicidal tendencies, among sufferers of headaches and migraines. A lack of sympathy and understanding among family, friends and work colleagues can greatly exacerbate any negative effects. Work, relationships and participation in social events or sports can all be adversely affected and, in extreme cases, the sufferer can end up out of work and socially isolated. Conversely, support and encouragement from those closely connected with the person is hugely important and can greatly enhance their ability to cope.

Getting help

In all the circumstances outlined above, two factors are critical: the ability to communicate and to seek help from others, and the ability to help oneself. If a sufferer is already feeling low or is actually depressed then self-help is less likely to take place. Fortunately, help from others is always available and a good place to begin is with the GP who, as well as providing medical care, may also refer the patient for onward professional psychological support or counselling. Talking to friends, family and people at work, especially one's immediate supervisor, is very important, since an apparently unsympathetic attitude may simply be caused by a lack of understanding. A further area of help lies with professional organisations; these can be contacted via the Internet and details of some are listed at the back of this book.

The importance of talking to people cannot be over-emphasised and it is through doing this that the route to self-help may be found. In this context, self-help means exploring any ways, however small and insignificant, that enable a sufferer to cope more effectively either with the pain itself or with its impact upon their life, and to exert a degree of control over their headaches.

Short pain inventory (SPI)

A relevant question at this stage is to ask if there is a means of measuring the extent to which a headache or migraine sufferer's life is being affected? There is a reliable and useful test called the short pain inventory (SPI) which measures this and which can be taken online for payment of a small fee at:

www.headachetest.co.uk

It includes a series of questions, which have been devised to accurately measure the effects of headache pain on everyday life. Some people may find it useful to try this, especially if they are finding it difficult to quantify effects for themselves.

Chapter 11
SECONDARY HEADACHES

Secondary headaches are uncommon, accounting for no more than 10% of all attacks at any particular time, and yet many people will experience a secondary headache at one time or another, generally in connection with a common, viral infection. Only a very small proportion of secondary headaches are attributable to a serious, life-threatening condition but many people have a disproportionate fear of headaches being caused by a severe malady such as a brain tumour.

In some cases, the secondary headache is the principle symptom of the condition that is causing it but it is more usual for it to be accompanied by a range of other symptoms. The illnesses and conditions that cause secondary headaches are described in some detail below, beginning with those that are most often involved.

Common cold

This frequently occurring, mild viral infection of the upper respiratory tract is often a cause of headaches. Other symptoms include inflammation of mucous membranes, streaming nose, watery eyes, sore throat, cough, fever, aches and pains affecting the face and possibly the joints. Headache arises as a result of the fever and slight dehydration that often accompanies the illness and can be alleviated by taking over-the-counter painkillers, drinking plenty of fluids, resting and staying warm until the symptoms subside.

Influenza, the flu

Influenza, or the flu, is a highly infectious, viral disease affecting the upper respiratory system. It causes headaches, fever, malaise, weakness, coughing, sneezing, sore throat, aches and pains in limbs and joints and loss of appetite. The symptoms can be severe and, rarely, the infection may prove fatal, especially in elderly people or those who are already ill and vulnerable. Influenza is of particular concern when it occurs in epidemics of a new strain to which the exposed population has little or no immunity. Headaches are associated with the fever and dehydration that accompanied the infection. An affected person should rest in bed, take over-the-counter painkillers and drink plenty of fluid. It may be necessary to continue to take analgesics for several days and it is important to keep warm and eat light meals. Flu symptoms can persist for two weeks although gradually improving and subsiding with time. It is not uncommon to continue to experience loss of appetite and tiredness for some time after other symptoms have subsided. Vaccination is available to protect the elderly and other vulnerable groups, offering some protection against certain viral strains and lessening severity in the event of infection.

Food poisoning

Food poisoning results from eating foods contaminated with any one of a number of different disease-causing bacteria. Food poisoning is most commonly caused by one of the following:

- By cross contamination, with organisms present on raw meat or chicken being transferred to cooked foods.
- By eating underdone food in which bacteria present have not been killed by the cooking process.
- By eating reheated food in which organisms have multiplied and have not been killed off by because the food has not reached a high enough temperature for a sufficient amount of time.
- By eating food that has been allowed to stand at room temperature for too long a time and so has become contaminated.

Symptoms include nausea and vomiting, diarrhoea, abdominal pains, headache and fever. The occurrence of headache is associated with the fever and dehydration caused by vomiting and diarrhoea.

Common types of food poisoning, named after the causal organism, include *Campylobacter*, *Salmonella* and *Staphylococcus aurea*. Less common ones are *Escherichia coli 0157*, *Listeria* and *Clostridium* (*Clostridium botulinum-botulism*). All types of food poisoning can be dangerous and sometimes fatal in the young, the old and those who are already in poor health or who have lowered immunity. *E. coli 0157* and botulism are particularly severe and there is risk of death or organ damage in those who survive a severe attack.

Strict food hygiene is essential to avoid the risk and there are a number of guidelines that should be followed:

- Wash hands thoroughly before and after handling food.
- Keep raw and cooked foods separate – raw meat should be wrapped and placed on a plate or in a suitable container on the bottom shelf of the refrigerator to ensure that there is no contact with other foods.
- Take especial care when handling raw chicken.

- Use separate chopping boards for preparing meat, fish and vegetables and wash all utensils thoroughly after use.
- Transfer cooked food to the refrigerator as soon as it has cooled. Do not leave it standing at room temperature for more than four hours. Meat and fish that has been defrosted should be placed in the refrigerator once thawed, unless it is being cooked immediately.
- Be especially vigilant when conditions are warm.
- Do not eat food containing raw egg.
- Do not eat unpasteurised dairy products. Buy soft cheeses such as Brie from a reputable source. Women should avoid eating certain dairy products during pregnancy.
- Cook food thoroughly and ensure that reheated food is heated right through.
- Observe manufacturer's recommendations.
- Observe 'sell-by' and 'eat-by' dates.
- Throw out any food that may be suspect without first sampling it.
- Do not allow pets near food preparation areas.
- Observe thorough hand hygiene at all times.
- Clean kitchen surfaces regularly.
- Change dish cloths and tea towels frequently, preferably every day.

Norovirus, the winter vomiting bug

Norovirus, or the winter vomiting bug, is usually short-lived but is a highly contagious infection of the gastrointestinal tract. The principle symptoms are projectile vomiting, nausea and diarrhoea but additionally, a significant proportion of people experience headache, fever, aches, pains, shivering (chills) and general tiredness and malaise. The infection is readily spread by personal contact or by handling objects contaminated with the virus and this is then inadvertently spread to the mouth. The illness passes easily from one family member to another or in any situation where people are gathered together, such as in hospitals, schools and work places. An infected person should stay at home to avoid spreading the illness to others and rest, drink as much fluid as possible, even if it is only sips of water and take over-the-counter painkilling medication, if necessary. Symptoms normally subside within 24 to 48 hours and the illness is not usually dangerous. However, vulnerable people such as the very young, the elderly and those with lowered immunity can be at risk and the principle danger is dehydration. Replacement fluids and electrolytes given intravenously may be required in extreme cases. Very stringent hygiene precautions should be observed in the event of an outbreak to try and control spread of the illness. Strict hand hygiene, avoiding shared use of items such as hand towels, thorough washing of utensils, such as cups, are all measures that should be adopted.

Dental problems

As might be expected, dental problems normally cause pain in the affected tooth or teeth or within the jaw. Occasionally, however, the pain is additionally experienced elsewhere as a headache and in this case it is known as 'referred pain'. In these circumstances it is probably unlikely that the headache will be felt on its own and appropriate dental treatment normally resolves the problem.

Temporomandibular joint dysfunction

The lower jaw is hinged to the skull on either side by means of the temporomandibular joint or TJM. Problems in the normal functioning of the TJM can be a cause of headaches and/or a trigger of migraine. The cause may relate to recent dental treatment such as fillings or a crown that is raised and has altered the bite but grinding of teeth (bruxism), usually during sleep, is sometimes implicated. Problems following dental treatment should be referred to a dentist and can usually be simply resolved. Teeth-grinding can be related to stress occurring during the day and medical advice should be sought if the problem is persistent.

Temporal arteritis, giant cell arteritis

Temporal arteritis, or giant cell arteritis, is poorly understood condition and a relatively common cause of headaches in those aged over 50 years. Women are at higher risk and it usually arises in people aged over 60 years. The arteries in the temple become inflamed and tender to the touch and throb visibly and this activity can be observed externally. The throbbing pain is centred over one eye but it is also sometimes felt elsewhere in the head and often, the scalp feels tender and sensitive. Chewing can exacerbate the problem and this is sometimes the cause of weight loss as eating becomes too painful. Without treatment there is a risk of blindness and hence an elderly person with these symptoms should always seek medical advice. Treatment, which is normally successful, involves long-term use of steroid drugs to relieve inflammation. Steroids are potent drugs and so patients must receive monitoring by a doctor who will check for adverse side effects.

Neck diseases and disorders

Wear and tear of the joints in the upper spine and neck causes inflammation and pain and is an occasional cause of headaches. Moving the head often exacerbates the pain and headache. Medical advice should be obtained and treatment includes use of anti-inflammatory and analgesic medication and possibly, physiotherapy and the wearing of a neck collar to provide support.

Chickenpox

Chickenpox is a highly infectious viral disease that usually affects children alone, in whom it is a relatively mild illness of fairly short duration. It causes fever, malaise and possibly headache before the appearance of a characteristic rash, comprising fluid-filled blisters. In adults, the illness is more severe, producing flu-like symptoms, fever, headache and malaise. In children, treatment is aimed at soothing the itching caused by the rash until the condition resolves. Adults may require medical treatment, depending upon severity of symptoms. The herpes zoster virus which is responsible for the infection remains dormant in the body for life, but may become activated at a later stage to produce an attack of shingles.

Shingles

Shingles affects the central nervous system, (specifically, the dorsal root ganglia) and follows the course of a nerve, causing severe pain and blisters on the skin over the affected part. Early symptoms include headache, chills, fever and malaise and the pain is often severe and debilitating. Shingles often strikes those with lowered immunity or people who have recently experienced stress and trauma. Medical treatment for the condition includes the use of steroid drugs, analgesics, corticosteroids and possibly, tranquillisers. Certain patients, especially those who are immuno-compromised, may require treatment with antiviral agents such as acyclovir.

Post-herpetic neuralgia

Following an attack of shingles, post-herpetic neuralgia, affecting various cranial nerves may arise. This often takes the form of a constant, deep-seated headache punctuated by intermittent episodes of acute, stabbing or 'needle-point' pain. Itching may accompany the pain. Various drugs are used in an attempt to alleviate this pain, which can be long-lasting and persist for several years. However, most patients gradually recover over a period of time or at least experience an improvement in their symptoms.

Trigeminal neuralgia, tic doloureux

Trigeminal neuralgia, or tic doloureux, affects the trigeminal nerve and it is thought that it is most usually caused by changes in fine blood vessels associated with nerve roots. The condition causes one-sided pain in the area of the face and head and this can be of a severe, burning, stabbing or cutting nature, sometimes described as resembling an electric shock. The pain lasts for between 2 and 120 seconds and women are three times more likely to be affected than men. The pain may be triggered by simple actions such as eating, face washing or cleaning teeth or by temperature changes. The skin of the face can become inflamed and the eye on the affected side is often watery and inflamed. The condition is highly debilitating and other symptoms such as facial tic, numbness or partial paralysis can occur as well as muscle wastage. The pain can be so severe that it interferes with sleeping and eating, and weight loss and lack of appetite are a recognised risk. Treatment includes the use of various drugs including analgesics and carbamazepine. If the condition proves intractable, injections to freeze the nerve or surgery to remove part of it may prove necessary.

German measles, rubella

German measles, or rubella, is a highly infectious viral disease that mainly affects children, in whom it produces an illness that is normally relatively mild. Early symptoms include headache, shivering, sore throat and a slight fever with the eventual appearance of a rash, comprising small pink spots. A further marked feature, although short-lived, is swelling of the neck. The rash usually disappears after about a week but the child remains infectious for another 3 to 4 days. Treatment consists of rest, ensuring a good intake of fluid, light meals and over-the-counter analgesics designed for children. Children in the UK are offered protection against the infection by immunisation with the MMR vaccine. German measles can cause foetal abnormalities in the early stages of pregnancy and for this reason young girls in the UK are again vaccinated against the virus around the age of 12 to 13 years. However, it is wise for a pregnant woman to avoid any known contact with the infection.

Measles

Measles is an extremely infectious viral disease that usually affects children and tends to occur in epidemics every 2 or 3 years. Preventative treatment in the form of the MMR vaccine is offered to all children in the UK to protect them against measles and its potentially serious or even fatal complications. However, due to fears of a link between vaccination and childhood autism, some parents have chosen not to allow their children to be vaccinated and for this reason, the incidence of measles has increased in recent years. Early symptoms include headache, high fever, coughing, sneezing and watering eyes. Small red spots with a white centre (known as Koplik's spots) may occur in the mouth, followed by the appearance of a characteristic rash of small red spots that may arise in groups. Any child suspected to have measles should be seen by a doctor to confirm the diagnosis. Emergency medical help should be sought in the event of the child developing a very high temperature, severe headache or earache or breathing difficulties. Complications can occur especially pneumonia and middle ear infection (and the latter can result in deafness). Also, brain inflammation (encephalitis) or meningitis can develop in the wake of measles infection and in a small number of children, death may occur. Vaccination protects children from the severe symptoms of measles and from its complications and it is in the child's best interests to be vaccinated in early childhood. No scientific evidence has been gathered to prove a link between MMR and autism. Adults who have not been immunised and who have not contracted measles during childhood are at risk from the infection and symptoms may be severe.

Scarlet fever, scarletina

Scarlet fever, or scarletina, is a bacterial infection in which the characteristic feature is a bright red skin rash. The illness mainly affects children and it is usually preceded by streptococcal throat infection. The causal organisms are erythrogenic toxins produced by haemolytic Group A streptococci. Although scarlet fever used to be a serious and feared illness of childhood responsible for many premature deaths, it is now generally mild and relatively rare, thanks to the use of antibiotics to treat the initial throat infection. It is rare in children aged less than 2 years and the most likely age group to contract the infection are children aged 2 to 10 years.

Symptoms appear after an incubation period of about 3 days and include a very high temperature, headache, chills, rapid pulse rate, extremely sore throat, vomiting, swollen, tender glands in the neck and throat. Within 24 hours, a bright red rash appears which feels like fine sand paper to the touch. The rash fades after about a week with peeling of the skin. When the illness is at its height, the tongue and face are usually a bright strawberry red colour although with a pale white ring around the mouth. Also, characteristically there are dark red lines in skin folds and creases. Treatment consists of bed rest, analgesics to deal with fever and pain and a course of antibiotics, either penicillin or erythromycin.

The child should be encouraged to drink plenty of fluids although this can be problematic if the throat continues to be sore. Usually, a child makes a complete recovery in a relatively short space of time. Complications are rare but include a throat abscess, ear infection, sinusitis, pneumonia, bronchopneumonia, rheumatic fever, septicaemia, meningitis, osteomyelitis (infection and inflammation of bones and bone marrow) and acute kidney failure. In rare cases, the infection can recur but if this happens it is caused by a different strain of bacteria (toxin) as one attack normally confers immunity.

Diabetes

Diabetes occurs in two main forms: Type 1, which arises in childhood and Type 2, which used to be a condition of middle age but is now affecting younger people. Type 2 diabetes is strongly correlated with diet and obesity. Both types are connected with a defect and imbalance in the metabolism of carbohydrates (sugars). There is an absence or imbalance in the production and release of the hormone, insulin (the substance responsible for regulating sugar levels in the blood), from the pancreas. Headaches can be associated with diabetes for two main reasons: the possible existence of hypertension and/or hypoglycaemia (low blood-sugar levels). Headaches are most likely to occur when diabetes is poorly controlled or prior to diagnosis, as it is known that many people have Type 2 diabetes without realising that this is the case. Diabetes is a serious condition carrying with it a risk of significant complications, including heart disease, kidney and eye disorders and wounds and ulcers on the lower limbs and feet that sometimes result in amputation. Type 2 diabetes is showing a worrying increase in incidence among younger adults and even adolescents and this is strongly linked to rising levels of obesity. It is especially important for anyone diagnosed with diabetes to make an effort to control their weight, to eat a healthy, fibre-rich diet and to adhere to the lifestyle and medication regime which they have been advised to follow. Sometimes, people affected by migraines who are later diagnosed with diabetes notice a lessening of headache incidence and severity. This is due to blood-sugar levels being properly controlled and it underlines the importance of vigilance in the treatment of diabetes.

Acute, narrow angle glaucoma , primary angle closure glaucoma

Acute, narrow angle glaucoma, or primary angle closure glaucoma, affects people who are middle-aged or elderly and symptoms may arise suddenly or be more intermittent and episodic in nature. They include a severe, throbbing pain around an eye and in the temple on that side, blurring of vision and vision disturbance, particularly seeing a halo of coloured light around a lamp. Also, nausea, vomiting and redness and inflammation of the eye may be present. The pupil becomes midrodilated and fixed and the eyeball is hard and tender, with the angle between the iris and cornea becoming closed. All symptoms are caused by the inability of fluid (aqueous humour) within the eye to drain normally, thus causing an acute build-up of pressure (ocular hypertension). If left untreated, there is damage to the retina and optic nerve leading to loss of sight. In the absence of painful, acute symptoms, diagnosis is suggested if a person reports seeing a coloured halo around lights. The condition necessitates emergency medical treatment, initially comprising administration of eye drops to reduce intra-ocular pressure and followed by surgery to restore drainage and prevent recurrence. It is not known exactly why the condition arises but inherited genetic factors, smoking and aging are the principle risks. Glaucoma can be detected by means of regular eye tests and these should take place every 3 years or more frequently, if a person is deemed to be at risk.

Hypertension, high blood pressure

Hypertension, or high blood pressure, is an increase over and above the normal range in the pressure exerted by the arterial blood circulation. It may be a condition in itself or a symptom of some other disorder or illness. Most forms of hypertension can present with few or no symptoms in the early stages and all forms appear to be more prevalent among Western populations.

Essential hypertension affects those in middle age, especially men aged over 40 years and most commonly between the ages of 50 and 60 years. In the later stages, or when symptoms arise, there may be headache present on awakening and this wears off gradually during the day only to return again in the evening. The headache is often felt in the back of the head and may be accompanied by ringing in the ears (tinnitus) and dizziness. Treatment involves lifestyle changes with regard to diet (a low-salt, low-fat diet is usually recommended), weight loss, if necessary, increased exercise and measures to reduce stress, if appropriate. Smoking should be avoided. Many anti-hypertensive drugs are available and one or more of these may be prescribed. They include beta-adrenoreceptor-blockers, thiazide diuretics, angiotensin inhibitors such as catopril, guanethidine and methyldopa.

Malignant hypertension can arise in younger people of either sex, producing symptoms similar to those described above and it is a medical emergency, requiring immediate treatment in hospital. In addition to the above symptoms, there is high diastolic pressure, often of rapid onset. Diastole is the point at which the heart relaxes between contractions (beats), when the ventricles (the large chambers) are filled with blood. Diastolic pressure is that which is exerted at this point and it should normally be low). Also, there is high intracranial pressure and this causes swelling of the first part of the optic nerve (the optic disc or papilla) – a condition known as papilloedema. Malignant hypertension causes damage to blood vessels in the brain, kidneys and heart and is fatal if not treated quickly. Death is often due to kidney failure.

Idiopathic intracranial hypertension is a relatively rare form of malignant hypertension that is especially likely to affect young women, especially those who are overweight or obese. There also appears to be a connection with taking the oral contraceptive pill and possibly certain other drug treatments. Symptoms include a headache that becomes gradually more severe and the cause is swelling of brain cells, leading to an increase in pressure within the skull. The reason why this occurs is not entirely understood. Diagnosis is made by means of a lumbar puncture to test the pressure of cerebrospinal fluid. Draining off some of the fluid often relieves the headache and the procedure may need to be repeated several times. Once again, this is an emergency condition requiring immediate treatment in hospital.

With early detection and treatment to bring pressure down, the risk of the development of serious complications of hypertension can be greatly reduced.

Sinusitis

Sinusitis is inflammation of a sinus (one of a number of air cavities present in the bones of the face and skull). Sinusitis usually refers to the sinuses in the face that are linked with the nasal passages of the nose. Hence the cause of the inflammation is often due to a spread of infection from the nose and there is usually an initial upper respiratory tract infection before sinusitis appears. Symptoms include headache, a stuffy, blocked nose and greenish, infected discharge, a feeling of heaviness and pain within the head and face and, possibly, sleep disruption. Treatment is by means of antibiotics and decongestants, usually in the form of nasal drops. Over-the-counter painkillers can be taken to relieve headache and pain. Rarely, if the condition persists and is severe, hospital admittance is needed and surgery to drain the affected sinus. Recurrence of sinusitis is quite common.

Antiphospholipid syndrome (ASS), 'sticky blood' syndrome, Hughes syndrome

ASS, or sticky blood syndrome, or Hughes syndrome, is an autoimmune condition characterised by an increased risk of blood-clotting disorders, such as deep vein thrombosis (DVT), pulmonary embolism, heart attack and stroke. It can affect both men and women but women are at greater risk of the condition. It is associated with the occurrence of headaches and migraine and, in women, with recurrent miscarriage. ASS may be either a primary condition or secondary, especially linked with the autoimmune disease called systemic lupus erythematosis (SLE).

Hughes Syndrome is caused by the abnormal production of antiphospholipid and other antibodies that attack the body's naturally occurring phospholipids and the proteins that bind to them. Phospholipids are essential molecules within the body and are especially found in the membranes that surround cells. ASS is responsible for around 15% of the incidence of recurrent miscarriage, especially that occurring after the first 12 weeks of pregnancy. Pregnant women are also at greater risk of developing complications, such as pre-eclampsia, if they have ASS. The syndrome has been found to be responsible for a significant proportion of heart attacks in younger adults and also DVT. Other symptoms that may arise include chorea (abnormal, jerky muscle movements), fits, memory lapses, confusion, blotchy skin rash (called livedo reticularis), giddiness, gastrointestinal disturbances, transient ischaemic attack (TIA), episodes mimicking multiple sclerosis and slight thrombocytopenia (low levels of blood platelets – the substances involved in clotting). ASS may be suspected following diagnosis of a circulatory disorder or repeated miscarriages, etc. It is diagnosed by means of a blood test to detect the antibodies and other tests may also be carried out. Treatment is by means of blood-thinning, anti-coagulant drugs, especially warfarin although this cannot be used during pregnancy. Some patients may be given other prepa-rations, including aspirin and heparin, according to individual need. Other lifestyle changes may be needed such as weight loss, exercise, adopting a healthy diet and giving up smoking to lessen the risk of heart attack or other serious circulatory event.

Aneurysm

An aneurysm is a balloon-like swelling in the wall of an artery that can occur when this becomes weakened or damaged in some way. Arteries in any part of the body can be affected but most commonly, aneurysm occurs in the brain (circle of Willis), aorta or the large arteries within the legs. Symptoms of a brain aneurysm include a throbbing headache, changes in the size of the pupils of the eyes, with one often being larger than the other and vision disturbance. There is a danger that the aneurysm will rupture causing bleeding (haemorrhage) with a risk of stroke and death. Hospital treatment involving surgery to remove or isolate the aneurysm and to restore the circulation by means of a graft or anastomosis (an artificial joining of the two undam-aged ends of the artery) is required. Anticoagulant drugs are likely to be needed along with other drugs, following surgery. Aneurysm may arise as a result of congenital weakness, espe-cially in the case of one affecting the circle of Willis (a ring of arteries supplying, and sited beneath the brain). Degenerative arterial disease (atherosclerosis) is another cause and this is a risk factor with increasing age. Some hardening of the arteries is, however, inevitable with aging. Other risk factors include a diet that is rich in animal fats, obesity, high blood pressure, a sedentary life style and smoking. All this emphasises the need to adopt a healthy life style at every stage in life and this includes taking regular exercise, eating a healthy low-fat, high-fibre diet and not smoking.

Stroke

A stroke describes the physical after-effects of an interruption in the blood supply to the brain and usually involves some degree of paralysis and damage of variable severity. The effects within the brain are secondary and the route cause lies within the heart and circulation. Causes include thrombosis, embolism and haemorrhage. Elderly adults of both sexes are at greater risk of stroke although younger people can also be affected. Symptoms vary according to the nature and severity of damage to the brain and may be gradual or sudden in onset. They include headache, loss of voluntary control over movement, numbness or tingling on one side of the body, mental confusion, loss of speech, confusion and vision disturbance. Also, the person may lose consciousness and he (or she) may appear flushed, breathe noisily, have a slow pulse rate and the pupils in each eye appear contracted unequally on either side. A stroke is a medical emergency requiring immediate admittance to hospital. Treatment is in the form of intensive care and support to maintain the patient in as stable a condition as possible. Some drugs may be administered, depending upon the nature of the stroke and they include antihypertensives, anticoagulants or heparin and nimodipine. A severe stroke is often fatal.

Patients who survive require physiotherapy to exercise paralysed limbs and all need a high level of support and encouragement to overcome the physical and cognitive disabilities that are the common aftermath of the condition. The cause of a stroke is usually atherosclerosis or hardening and narrowing of the arteries, which occurs with increasing age. This can result in blockage of an artery by a blood clot (thrombosis), resulting in an interruption in the blood flow to the brain. There may be an embolism in which a clot or plug of blood is carried from the heart or an artery to lodge in a blood vessel within the brain and so cause the interruption in the blood supply. A further cause is a brain haemorrhage with a sudden bleed that may have catastrophic results. In younger people, the cause is usually a ruptured aneurysm that has arisen due to an unsuspected congenital weakness, causing a *subarachnoid haemorrhage*.

Subarachnoid haemorrhage

Subarachnoid haemorrhage is bleeding into the subarachnoid space of the brain. This space lies between two of the membranes or meninges that cover the brain, called the arachnoid and the pia mater membranes. The space usually contains cerebrospinal fluid. Symptoms include a sudden and very severe headache, nausea and vomiting, dizziness, fainting and coma. Erratic heartbeat and breathing and seizures may also occur. Within 24 hours, the person develops a stiff neck and other muscle and reflex responses (called Kernig's sign and Babinski's sign). During the first few days after the bleeding, there continues to be a headache, confusion and a raised temperature. There may be one-sided paralysis (hemiplegia). The condition requires emergency medical treatment in hospital and there is a risk of stroke and death. Following admittance to hospital, diagnostic tests and scans are performed to determine the nature of the haemorrhage. The outlook is best for patients who are well enough to undergo surgery during the first 72 hours. A majority of patients survive a first subarachnoid haemorrhage but there is a risk of recurrence, especially within the first few weeks. Surgery reduces the risk of a subsequent haemorrhage. Patients may be left with residual brain damage and there can be some degree of paralysis, muscular weakness, confusion and speech difficulties. Hence recovery and rehabilitation can take some time and the person may not recover to the way he (or she) was before the bleed. The commonest cause is head injury but others include a ruptured aneurysm with atherosclerosis and hypertension being contributory factors. Rarely, bleeding may be caused by the presence of an arteriovenous malformation (AVM). Following a subarachnoid haemorrhage, there is a risk of raised intracranial pressure and this can be a cause of further headaches and hydrocephalus (an abnormal collection of cerebrospinal fluid within the skull).

Subdural haemorrhage, subdural haematoma, acute and chronic

Acute and chronic subdural haemorrhage, or subdural haematoma, is bleeding that takes place within the space between two of the membranes (meninges) that surround the brain, causing a collection or clot of blood to form, known as a haematoma. The membranes involved are called the dura mater, the outer membrane and the arachnoid mater, a middle layer of tissue.

An acute subdural haematoma is a common occurrence following a serious head injury and arises soon after the trauma has been sustained. Symptoms include headache, confusion, drowsiness, irritability and it is likely that the person may soon become unconscious. There is a risk of coma and death and the person requires immediate medical treatment, probably including emergency surgery.

A chronic subdural haematoma may occur some weeks after a seemingly trivial blow to the head and there may be a delay in the onset of symptoms. These include worsening headaches that arise each day, periods of drowsiness and confusion and one-sided muscular weakness. The person requires emergency medical treatment and, following admittance to hospital, diagnostic tests and scans are carried out to reveal the exact nature and location of the clot. Surgery is then needed to remove the clot and relieve the pressure on the brain that is responsible for the symptoms. Once the pressure is relieved, the brain may slowly recover but there can be degrees of permanent damage and disability and possibly, continuing headaches. Surgery is not always successful and there is a risk of death or severe brain damage and permanent disability. Older people are at greatest risk of a bleed of this nature but also younger ones with a history of alcohol abuse.

Arteriovenous malformation of the brain (AVM)

An AVM is a rarely occurring, abnormal development of tangled veins that can occur in any part of the body but more often within the brain. An AVM develops when the capillaries (fine, threadlike blood vessels) that usually act as a physical, intervening network between arteries and veins are absent for some reason. Blood in arteries flows at a much higher pressure than that in veins because it is pumped through the vessels by the heart. Arteries possess relatively thick, muscular walls to cope with this while those of veins are comparatively thin and weak. The capillary network normally dissipates the difference but in its absence, the blood received by the veins is at a much higher than normal pressure. The veins respond by expanding to form the tangled mass of an AVM. Brain AVMs are rare, being diagnosed in 1 in every 100,000 people, usually in those aged over 40 years and the underlying cause of the abnormality remains unknown. They vary in size and location within the skull and are not a part of brain tissue as such but of its blood supply. When an AVM occurs within the dura (the outer, fibrous membrane surrounding the brain), it is called a dural fistula. It is thought that brain AVMs may be present at birth but that they undergo change and development during the course of a person's lifetime. The main risk that is posed by an AVM is the potential for rupture and haemorrhage (*see* **Subarachnoid haemorrhage** on page 81 and **Subdural haemorrhage** on page 82). About a fifth of those with a brain AVM have no symptoms and the abnormality is discovered during investigations into some other condition. In 50% of cases, the AVM is found to be the cause of a brain haemorrhage and it is also a cause of epileptic seizures. It is a matter of debate as to whether brain AVMs are a direct cause of headaches or migraines and further research may help to establish whether this is the case.

Concussion

Concussion describes a state that may follow a blow to the head and it arises when the brain has suffered a degree of trauma and bruising. In all cases, there is a loss of consciousness but this varies in degree and may be partial or complete. Symptoms vary in severity and reflect, to some extent, the force of the blow. They include headache, dizziness, confusion, drowsiness and tiredness if concussion is mild but if severe, the person may lapse into unconsciousness and remain in this state for a variable period of time. It may be possible to partially arouse the person but he (or she) is then extremely irritable and cannot answer questions coherently and soon becomes unconscious once again. When the person finally comes out of unconsciousness, a severe headache is often present accompanied by irritability and extreme tiredness and these symptoms can persist for some time. Commonly, there is little or no memory of the events surrounding the blow to the head. A person with concussion requires admittance to hospital for close monitoring and possibly scans to ascertain if there has been any damage. There is a danger of bleeding (see **Subarachnoid haemorrhage** and **Subdural haemorrhage**) that may result in death or severe brain damage. While unconsciousness persists the patient remains hospitalised and even in mild cases, there is a need for ongoing observation of the person who will need to rest until headache and tiredness subside – a process that may take some time. The cause of concussion is a compression wave initiated by the blow to the head and this momentarily interrupts the blood supply to the brain. In mild cases most people eventually make a good recovery but there may be headaches, irritability, difficulty in concentrating and forgetfulness that persists for several months.

Meningitis

Meningitis is inflammation of the meninges, which are the membranes that surround the brain and spinal cord. The cause is either *bacterial* or *viral* infection and meningitis can arise as a complication of other infectious diseases including Lyme disease, leptospirosis, typhoid fever and typhus.

Bacterial meningitis is the most dangerous and potentially fatal form and it may be of rapid onset, causing a person to become very seriously ill over a period of hours. In other cases, the illness develops over 1 to 2 days and sometimes, acute meningitis develops to become a chronic form and this can cause severe brain damage. Bacterial meningitis is less common than the viral form of the illness but in all cases, admittance to hospital for emergency medical treatment at an early stage offers the best chance for recovery. Symptoms include a severe headache, a stiff, painful neck, a characteristic red/purplish rash with spots or bruising that remains when pressed with a glass, confusion, drowsiness, rapid breathing, vomiting, fever with high temperature but cold hands and feet, muscle and joint pains, abdominal pains and possibly diarrhoea and sensitivity to light. Coma and death may follow rapidly, in some cases. Septicaemia or blood poisoning, characterised by cold hands and feet, an unusual skin colour, high fever and leg pains can be an early indication of meningitis, especially in children. In infants, there may be refusal to feed, high temperature, vomiting, whimpering/moaning crying, fretfulness, dislike of being picked up, fits, retraction of neck and back arching, bulging fontanelle, lethargy and difficulty in wakening up, blank facial expression, paleness and itchiness. Infants are at risk of serious complications and death.

Viral meningitis produces symptoms that are generally less severe and these include headache, high fever, drowsiness, malaise, aches and pains, abdominal effects and in severe cases, vision disturbance, muscle weakness, partial paralysis, partial loss of ability to speak and fits. In some very rare cases, coma and death can occur. Although most patients recover, some people suffer from longer term hearing loss or memory impairment, and headaches, depression and fatigue may be present for some considerable time. Bacterial meningitis is treated with intensive intravenous antibiotics and sulphonamide drugs and the sooner these are started, the better the chances of recovery. Intravenous fluids and electrolytes are also likely to be administered. Viral meningitis requires good nursing care and admittance to hospital may not be necessary, depending upon severity. Some patients require more intensive treatment with antiviral drugs such as acyclovir, given intravenously.

Three types of bacteria are responsible for most cases of bacterial meningitis and these are: *Neisseria meningitides*, (meningococcus), *Streptococcus pneumoniae*, (pneumococcus) and *Haemophilus influenzae type b*, (Hib). In the UK, the first two bacteria are usually involved with meningococcal infection most common among infants and pneumococcal infection more usual in adults. Other causal bacteria include *E.coli*, *Mycobacterium tuberculosis* and Group B *Streptococcus*. Meningococcus and certain other types occur naturally at the back of the nose and throat with a certain proportion of the population harbouring the organisms at any one time without becoming ill themselves. The bacteria are passed on through close contact, kissing, sneezing or coughing. Viruses that may cause meningitis include echo/enteroviruses, Coxsackie, varicella zoster, polio virus, herpes simplex, mumps virus. Viral meningitis is most prevalent among young people in schools and colleges. Routine vaccination is carried out in the UK to immunise children against Hib and meningococcus C, in the form of the Men C vaccination.

Glandular fever, infectious mononucleosis

Glandular fever, or infectious mononucleosis, is an infectious, viral illness caused by the Epstein Barr virus and it usually arises in adolescents and young adults of both sexes. There is widespread swelling of lymph nodes in the neck, armpits and groin and symptoms include headache, loss of appetite, general malaise and fatigue. The liver and spleen may become enlarged and jaundice can occasionally develop. A person showing symptoms of glandular fever should be seen by a doctor to confirm diagnosis and this is made by means of a blood test. Treatment consists of bed rest and taking over-the-counter painkilling medication, as advised by a doctor. It is important to drink plenty of fluids and eat as good a balanced diet as appetite allows. Complications rarely arise but include a ruptured spleen which requires emergency admittance to hospital and the surgical removal of this organ. Recovery from glandular fever can be prolonged with continuing excessive fatigue and malaise being a relatively common experience. The condition is especially likely to occur in young people living in conditions where they are in close proximity such as in university halls of residence, boarding schools or military establishments. It is thought that young people are vulnerable due to their having an immature immune system compared to that of adults.

Myalgic encephalopathy/encephalomyelitis (ME), chronic fatigue syndrome (CFS), post-viral fatigue syndrome (PVS)

ME, or chronic fatigue syndrome (CFS), or post-viral fatigue syndrome (PVS), is a disorder that has been the subject of considerable debate and one that is characterised by extreme fatigue accompanied by a range of other symptoms. The fatigue is chronic and persistent, is not related to levels of physical activity and is not relieved by rest. Other symptoms include chronic headaches, muscle and joint pains and aches, lapses in memory and ability to concentrate, depression, anxiety, panic attacks, sleep disturbances, insomnia and general malaise. Digestive disturbances, nausea, sensitivity to noise and light and vision disturbance are further frequent symptoms. Some people develop a heightened sensitivity to touch or may experience a crawling sensation in the skin.

A person affected by ME finds it impossible to function normally although there is no obvious sign of disease or malady. Normal patterns of work and activity become impossible and those affected can suffer a great deal of social isolation alongside their physical symptoms. ME is thought to arise following a viral infection and a number of viruses have been implicated and occur in conjunction with an altered or disordered immune response. Enteroviruses (those that enter via the gut), the Epstein Barr virus (see **Glandular fever** on page 87) and some others are possibly involved. A different type of organism called mycoplasma has also been implicated. There is no specific treatment for ME but bed rest is usually essential and other medication to relieve aches, pains and headaches may be helpful. The patient requires considerable emotional support from those closely involved and may benefit from psychological and complementary therapies, particularly to help cope with depression. Young patients are likely to require educational support in the longer term to help them make up for lost schooling. Recovery from ME can be prolonged but the majority of those affected improve slowly and gradually with time, although this can take months or even 2 to 3 years, in some cases and following recovery, the person may always be prone to tiredness.

Fibromyalgia (FMS)

Fibromyalgia is a chronic illness with around 15,000 people each year in the UK being newly diagnosed with this condition. It affects about 1 in every 100 people at some stage during their lifetime and 90% of sufferers are women. Characteristically, there are widespread aches and pains in joints, muscles and ligaments arising in any part of the body but especially in the lower limbs, feet, back, shoulders and neck. The pains often move about and are frequently worse in the morning, improve during the day and become more severe again at night. Specific tender spots, experienced as pain when the skin is lightly pressed are a further characteristic feature and the areas most commonly involved are the neck, hips, elbows and knees. The pains experienced may be burning, throbbing or aching in nature. It is quite common for analgesic medication to be of limited effect in relieving the aches and pains associated with fibromyalgia. Extreme fatigue can be experienced although this varies in severity but quite frequently the person awakes feeling exhausted even following a good night's sleep. Other common symptoms include chronic headache, facial pain, malaise, digestive disturbances, nausea, poor concentration and memory lapses, sleep disturbance, numbness and/or tingling sensations in the feet and hands (called paresthesia), restless legs, especially at night in bed, dry mouth and/or skin and eyes and, in women, painful periods and pain with intercourse.

Psychological symptoms of anxiety and depression are common and severity of symptoms may vary with levels of daily activity and environmental and emotional factors such as stress. The condition can show a relapsing pattern with periods when symptoms greatly improve or disappear entirely and there are evident similarities with ME. Various causes have been suggested although the exact cause of the condition remains unknown and a combination of factors may be involved. However, research has revealed that sufferers have a lowered level of the hormone serotonin and this substance is known to play a role in pain and sleep regulation and is a significant factor in the occurrence of certain types of primary headache. Treatment may be multifaceted, including rest, the use of medication and psychological and complementary therapies. Emotional support is very important and an affected person should be encouraged to lead as normal a life as the condition allows. A good, healthy diet and taking exercise, as far as strength permits, are all recommended to help relieve the condition.

Lyme disease

Lyme disease is a tick-borne bacterial infection caused by the spirochaete bacterium, *Borellia burgdorfen*. The parasitic ticks that carry the organism are widespread among wild animals, such as deer, and at a certain stage in the life cycle are to be found among vegetation, from where they readily attach themselves to the body of any passing mammal. Dogs often pick up ticks while being walked in the countryside but the insects also latch onto people and it is thought that the mild winters of recent years have favoured a rise in their number. An increasing number of people are being affected and ticks have now been found in vegetation in town gardens. Not all ticks carry the infective organism but the incidence of diagnosed cases of Lyme disease is rising and it is thought that many more people may be affected unawares.

The ticks are tiny, black insects that can be hard to spot with the naked eye, especially when they first become attached. If left undisturbed, the insect enlarges as it gorges on blood and eventually drops off, when ready to complete its life cycle. The bite causes a small, red lump or papule and this usually eventually forms a scab on the surface of the skin. Infection with Lyme disease occurs when the organism passes into the blood supply and an early sign may be a red ring around the site of the bite. The area then expands and reddens and may become enlarged and further skin lesions may appear.

Other symptoms include headache, fever, malaise, chills, aches and pains in the neck and muscles and fatigue. Nausea, vomiting, a sore throat and enlargement of the lymph glands and spleen may also occur. A chronic form of Lyme disease can develop weeks, months or even years after the initial infection causing bouts of periodic illness. In about half of all cases, arthritic joint pain and swelling occurs, especially affecting the knee and this usually arises after a period of weeks or months following initial infection. Less commonly, but in a similar time scale, there can be inflammation and enlargement of the heart with conduction disorders and/or effects on the central nervous system. Aseptic meningitis and Bell's Palsy are recognised complications of Lyme disease affecting the central nervous system. Chronic fatigue, muscular aches and pains, poor concentration and memory lapses are further potential consequences. If you notice a skin lesion and suspect a tick bite, you should seek medical advice, especially in the event of inflammation or flu-like symptoms. Diagnosis is by means of a blood test to detect infection and a course of antibiotics kills the bacteria and prevents future complications from arising. In chronic cases following a delayed diagnosis, medication to alleviate symptoms along with other appropriate treatments are required.

Anyone working outdoors or taking part in leisure activities in the countryside should be aware of the risks of tick bites and take simple precautions. These include wearing clothing that covers the flesh – especially long trousers rather than shorts and boots or stout shoes instead of open sandals. Trouser bottoms should be tucked into socks to prevent the insects from attaching to the ankles. Following a day out, the skin should be carefully examined for the presence of ticks. It is usually possible to remove a tick quite easily while it is small and has not become attached too firmly but it is essential that the insect's mouth parts do not remain embedded in the skin. If there is any doubt about this, it is best to seek medical advice.

Cat scratch fever

Cat scratch fever is a mild fever of viral origin that causes swelling of the lymph glands and a slight infection at the site of the scratch or puncture wound. Other symptoms include headache and feverishness, mild discomfort and malaise. Treatment involves rest until symptoms subside, along with taking over-the-counter analgesic medication, as required and ensuring a good fluid intake. Medical treatment is usually not necessary unless symptoms worsen or in the event of an abscess developing at the site of the wound. Recovery normally takes place quickly, within a few days. The cause is a virus that enters the blood stream via a scratch from a pet cat or thorn or splinter. Cat scratches are responsible for about half of all cases of the infection.

Encephalitis

Encephalitis is inflammation and swelling of the brain. It is caused either directly by a viral infection of the brain or results from an autoimmune disorder when, following infection by a virus, the body's immune system reacts abnormally and attacks the tissues of the central nervous system. This condition is called autoimmune encephalitis or post-infectious encephalitis and it is a more common form of the illness. True viral encephalitis is very rare, affecting about 4 in every 100,000 people each year in the UK. If the meninges (the membranes surrounding the brain and spinal cord) are also involved, the condition is more correctly termed *meningoencephalitis*. If the spinal cord is affected as well as the brain, then the illness is called *encephalomyelitis*.

Encephalitis can arise suddenly or show a more insidious pattern of onset and symptoms vary from mild to extremely severe and fatal. Early symptoms may mimic those of flu and they include severe headache, fever, stiff neck and back, fits, confusion, drowsiness that may deepen into coma, irritability, irrational behaviour, loss of ability to speak, lack of coordination, photosensitivity and memory lapses. A person suffering from encephalitis needs emergency treatment in hospital and intensive nursing care. Of initial concern is to reduce the pressure on the brain. Encephalitis is a serious illness and can be fatal and even after recovery, there can be problems caused by residual brain damage. Also, headaches, irritability, lack of concentration and extreme fatigue quite commonly persist for some time. Many viruses can cause encephalitis including rubella (German measles), Epstein Barr (glandular fever), influenza, chickenpox (varicella), measles (rubeola), poliovirus, herpes simplex, HIV, toxoplasmosis and cytomegalovirus. Arboviruses are carried by ticks and mosquitoes and are responsible for certain types of encephalitis in various parts of the world, including West Nile fever and Japanese encephalitis.

Heatstroke, heat hyperpyrexia

Heatstroke, or heat hyperpyrexia, is a severe condition that results from overexposure of the body to excessive heat. Symptoms include failure of sweating and all temperature regulation, severe headache, muscle cramps, hot dry skin and high body temperature. There is a rapid heartbeat and eventual loss of consciousness, coma and death and this can follow quite quickly. The person requires immediate emergency attention to save life and admittance to hospital. The body is overheated and must be cooled immediately by sponging or immersion in cool water and fanning. The body may be wrapped in wet sheets. Once the temperature has returned to normal, the person should be dried and wrapped in a dry blanket. When consciousness returns, drinks and salt solutions are needed or may have to be given intravenously. The cause of the symptoms is loss of fluid and salt through excessive sweating leading to disruption of the salt/water balance, lowered blood volume, metabolic disturbance and shock. Preventative measures include taking enough time for acclimatisation to the heat and increasing fluid intake. People who are required to carry out hard, physical work need to drink salt solutions to compensate for the loss that occurs with profuse sweating.

Brain tumour

A brain tumour is a growth of abnormal cells within the brain or meninges (membranes) and it may be either *benign* or *malignant* (cancerous). Brain tumours are rare and vary in severity but all are serious conditions that may prove fatal. A malignant brain tumour is classed as either *primary* (one that has grown in the brain in the absence of any cancer elsewhere in the body) or *secondary* (one that has arisen in the brain as a result of cancerous cells being transported in the blood circulation from a primary tumour in a different organ such as the breast). Brain tumours are more common in adults but ones that occur in children may, in some cases, be congenital. Usually, the cause of any particular tumour is unknown.

Symptoms vary according to the precise location of the tumour but early ones are nearly always associated with a rise in intracranial pressure caused by the tumour growing and pressing upon the brain. They include a headache which is often worse on first awakening and is exacerbated by exertion or coughing, nausea, vomiting, dizziness, loss of balance and coordination, one-sided weakness/numbness, fits, confusion and changes in cognitive ability, altered senses (of taste and smell), problems with speech or ability to read and write, personality changes and vision disturbance. Sometimes a tumour in a particular site produces a set of symptoms that lead to its presence being suspected but quite often, the situation may not be clear cut and diagnosis may only be made after a number of tests have been carried out and a brain scan obtained.

Treatment depends upon the location and nature of the tumour and the approach adopted will vary in each case. Quite often, steroid drugs are given on admittance to hospital to reduce swelling and inflammation in the brain and this usually brings about an improvement in debilitating headache pain and makes the person feel better, in the short term. There are three treatment options and these may be used either alone or more often, in combination: surgery, radiotherapy and chemotherapy. Before any type of brain surgery is performed, a cost/benefit evaluation has to be made as to how much damage the procedure itself might cause. Surgery is more likely to be carried out if the tumour is accessible and if there is a good chance that most, if not all of it, can be removed. Advances in all forms of treatment have meant that more brain tumours can be treated now than was the case in the past. Although treatment is not always curative, it is normally expected that it will enhance quality of life and hopefully also extend the likely survival period. In some cases of slow-growing, benign brain tumour the best option may be monitoring rather than intervention, depending upon severity of symptoms.

Q fever

Q fever is a relatively rare, bacterial infection that can be transmitted to humans through close contact with infected farm animals. The causal bacteria are called *Coxiella burnetti* and they are commonly found in sheep, goats and cattle in which they do not produce illness, although they can be responsible for stillbirth. About 70 cases are diagnosed annually in the UK but it is thought that many more may go unreported as the illness can be mild in some people or even produce no symptoms. The organism is present in the milk, urine, faeces and blood of infected animals and is particularly to be found in the placenta after calving or lambing. Once outside the body of the animal, the bacteria can survive for several months if temperatures are relatively mild. The organism can be transmitted by breathing in infected particles or by touching anything contaminated with infected animal fluids or waste and then raising the hands to the mouth, or the organisms may gain access into the bloodstream via uncovered cuts or grazes. The bacteria cannot be transmitted directly from person to person and those most at risk are farmers and veterinary staff, especially during calving and lambing, and people who work in abattoirs or animal rescue establishments.

Symptoms, if present, arise 2 to 3 weeks after exposure and produce a flu-like illness with headaches, fever, muscle and joint pains, malaise, breathing difficulty and a cough being commonly present. Symptoms sometimes show a pattern of very rapid onset. The illness persists for about 2 weeks but in some people, a chronic form can arise and in this case, symptoms may continue for 6 months or more. Also, severe symptoms of Q fever can occasionally recur and flare up several years after the initial infection. Pregnant women are at particular risk, both with regard to their own health and that of their unborn child. A woman who is pregnant should avoid close contact with farm animals especially any that have just given birth.

Those diagnosed with the illness may be treated by means of antibiotics, especially tetracycline and doxycycline, although these are less effective for the chronic form of the condition. Bed rest and drinking plenty of fluids and taking over-the-counter analgesic medication help to relieve symptoms. A protective vaccine is available for workers identified as being at risk and strict standards of animal welfare and hygiene practices (strict hand washing, dust extraction measures, etc) also help to reduce the likelihood of infection.

Phaeochromocytoma

Phaeochromocytoma is a tumour of an adrenal gland (one of a pair of endocrine or hormone-secreting glands situated above each kidney). The tumour is normally benign (non-cancerous) and is usually located in the inner part of the gland, known as the medulla. It is usually just a few centimetres in diameter but rarely can grow to be a considerable size and weight. It is most likely to occur in adults aged 30 to 50 years. The tumour causes an excess production of the adrenal hormones, adrenaline and noradrenaline and this imbalance is the cause of many of the symptoms.

Symptoms include hypertension, headache, nausea, vomiting, weight loss, palpitations, clammy skin, nervousness, anxiety, tachycardia (rapid heartbeat rate), fainting, sweating, disturbance of vision, and sudden drop in blood pressure when rising up from a prone position. Analysis of urine samples for the presence of catecholamines (breakdown products of adrenal hormones) and scans confirm the diagnosis.

Treatment involves admittance to hospital for drug therapy prior to surgical removal of the tumour. There is a risk of death through stroke or circulatory disorder associated with the hypertension that is a significant factor in phaeochromocytoma and the cause of headache in this condition.

Polycythaemia rubra vera, secondary polycythaemia

Polycythaemia is an excessive production of red blood cells in the blood. Primary polycythaemia, or polycythaemia rubra vera, is a rare disorder in which red blood cells, white blood cells and platelets are all produced in excessive amounts. Secondary polycythaemia arises as a result of some other disorder.

Symptoms include headache, weariness, breathlessness, disturbance of vision, itching, flushed skin, bleeding and enlargement of the spleen. Complications may arise including symptoms of peptic ulcer, pain in the bones, thrombosis, gout, kidney stones and liver disorder. Treatment may involve admittance to hospital for phlebotomy (the incision of a vein to allow blood to be collected – now usually known as venesection). Also, chemotherapy with cytotoxic drugs and radiotherapy with radioactive phosphate may be required.

Treatment is tailored to the individual needs of the patient and one or more methods may be needed, depending upon response. Also, other drugs such as aspirin and other analgesic drugs along with medication to relieve itching may be needed. Primary polycythaemia is incurable although the symptoms can be relieved and the cause is unknown. Secondary polycythaemia is curable if the underlying disorder is amenable to treatment. Smoking, living at high altitude for an extended period, chronic lung disease, or tumours of the brain, liver, kidney or uterus are all recognised risk factors. There is a risk of death from thrombosis, bone marrow failure or haemorrhage and an increased likelihood of the development of leukaemia.

Malaria

Malaria is a feverish infection caused by minute parasites in the blood, characterised by recurring bouts of fever. The cause is infection with any one of four types of protozoan organisms, all of which belong to the genus *Plasmodium*, namely *P. falciparium*, *P. malariae*, *P. vivax* and *P. ovale*. These organisms complete a stage of their lifestyle within female anopheles mosquitoes and the insects acquire the parasites by feeding on the blood of an infected person. The parasites are then passed on to new human hosts when the mosquitoes next bite in order to feed. Mosquitoes feed by piercing a minute vein in the skin and in this way the parasites gain access to the blood circulation and lodge in the liver where they multiply. Returning to the bloodstream they invade more and more red blood cells, eventually causing these to enlarge and rupture.

Depending upon the species of parasite, symptoms develop between 1 to 4 weeks following a bite from an infective mosquito. Before the onset of the attack, the person may feel somewhat unwell for 1 or 2 days and typically there are three stages to the illness, although these may not always be apparent. An initial 'cold stage' is characterised by extreme shivering and feeling excessively chilled, even though the person has a high temperature. After about an hour, this is followed by the 'hot stage' in which the temperature rises even higher and there is a burning fever, severe headache, nausea, giddiness, pain and possible delirium. The final, 'sweating stage' is characterised by profuse sweating and a fall in temperature. The aches and pains and headache subside and the person feels better although he (or she) is left in a weakened state. There is then a lapse of a few hours, (the period varying according to the species of parasite), before the next attack and repeat of symptoms. There may be widespread destruction of red blood cells, especially with repeated recurrent bouts of malaria and the disease can become chronic and leave the patient with severe anaemia. More usually, even in the absence of treatment, the number of parasites in the blood falls to a low level until there is no recurrence of symptoms. However, the parasites can also become active again and multiply to produce further attacks of fever. Fever bouts correspond with the rupturing of red blood cells and the released parasites then go on to invade fresh blood cells. If the infective organism is *P. vivax* or *P. ovale*, it may persist within the liver for a very long time. There is a risk of death caused by the high fever of a malarial attack and the parasites may become so numerous as to block small blood vessels within the brain (*cerebral malaria*) and this is also a cause of mortality. A further dangerous complication is blackwater fever, characterised by high fever, severe anaemia and a huge destruction of red blood cells, leading to loss of haemoglobin (oxygen-carrying red pigment in blood) in urine. Malaria is at its most dangerous in people who are malnourished, immuno-compromised or who are very young or old. Also, in those who do not receive adequate treatment so that some of the parasites survive.

Complete bed rest and good intake of fluids is very important, along with antimalarial drugs such as chloroquinine that may need to be given intravenously. Treatment in hospital is usually required and is essential for those who are very ill. Malaria cannot be contracted in the UK at the present time although there is increasing concern that global warming may enable the malarial mosquito to extend its range further north. Various preventative drugs are available and anyone contemplating travel to a country where malaria is prevalent should take medical advice as to which of these is appropriate. A course of drugs should be taken within a certain time period before departure but although these preparations offer some protection, they may not be entirely effective against infection. Other precautions include sleeping beneath mosquito netting and the vigilant application of effective insect repellent lotion to the skin.

Toxic shock syndrome (TSS)

Toxic shock syndrome is a rarely occurring state of acute shock due to a form of blood poisoning caused by toxins (poisons) produced by streptococcal or staphylococcal bacteria. Children and young adults are at greater risk of developing TSS and it is believed that this is due to the immune system being relatively more immature and less effective in this age group. Streptococcal TSS is more common than staphylococcal TSS and it is more difficult to treat and has a higher rate of mortality. It arises when the bacteria gain access to the blood stream either via a wound (possibly a surgical wound) or during an infection such as chickenpox, as a result of scratching of spots – although this is rare. The bacteria then produce the toxins that are responsible for TSS although why this occurs in some circumstances and not in others is not clear. Staphylococcal bacteria produce their toxins at the body's surface and do not require initial access to the bloodstream. TSS from this cause can arise in young women during menstruation, especially if tampons are being used but also, in both sexes, following on from infections such as flu or boils on the skin, burns, wounds (including surgical) and abrasions.

Symptoms include sudden high fever, severe headache, a red skin rash, anxiety, diarrhoea, confusion, behavioural changes, thirst and a fall in blood pressure.

In the case of TSS in a young woman during menstruation, removing the tampon may avert more severe symptoms. If tampons are being used and there is sudden onset of high fever and a rash, it is advised to remove the tampon immediately before seeking further medical help. A person suffering from TSS needs to be admitted to hospital for emergency medical treatment, monitoring and intensive nursing care. Oxygen must first be given to a shocked patient and also intravenous fluids to restore blood volume and elevate blood pressure. High doses of intravenous antibiotics, especially clindamycin are needed and immunoglobulins administered by the same route help to neutralise the bacterial toxins. Early treatment offers the best chance of the patient making a full recovery but TSS can be fatal in some cases. There are about five cases of TSS associated with tampon use each year. Women should wash their hands before inserting a tampon, use the lowest possible absorbency, change tampons frequently and occasionally use a sanitary towel instead. It is particularly important to remember to remove the last tampon used at the end of the period.

Leptospirosis

Leptospirosis is an acute infection caused by bacteria belonging to the genus *Leptospira*. The causal organisms are found in the urine of many animals including cattle, foxes and rats. Farmers, veterinarians, sewage/waste-water workers, fish-farm workers, etc, are all at greater occupational risk as are persons who swim in contaminated water. Pregnant women are at greater risk of miscarriage, even after recovery from the infection. One particular species of the organism, *L. icterohaemorrhagiae*, is found in the urine of rats and is responsible for Weil's disease.

In the early stages, symptoms mimic those of flu and include intense throbbing headache with pain over the eye, fever, chills, shivering, aches and pains in muscles and joints, diarrhoea and digestive upset, enlargement of lymph nodes, cough, mental disturbances, internal bleeding and palpitations. The kidneys may be involved and also the liver, causing severe damage and jaundice, or the central nervous system, with a risk of meningitis.

Treatment involves courses of antibiotics particularly penicillin, streptomycin, erythromycin or tetracyclines and these must be started as soon as possible, within a week of the onset of symptoms. Admittance to hospital for intravenous antibiotic treatment and supportive nursing is essential for those who are seriously ill. If the major organs have become involved, antibiotic treatment is less effective and occasionally an effect called the Jarisch-Herxheimer reaction is observed, caused by sudden release of toxins from dying bacteria. Symptoms of this include severe headache, chills and muscular pains. In most cases, symptoms are mild and there is a good recovery but there is a risk of more severe complications, as outlined above. To prevent infection, do not enter or swim in water that may be contaminated. Bacteria can gain access through skin cuts and abrasions but also via the mucous membranes that line the mouth and nose – hence the risk posed by swimming. Those whose occupation puts them at risk should exercise extreme vigilance, including the wearing of protective clothing and particularly, stringent hand hygiene measures.

Rat bite fever

Two types of infection producing similar symptoms both of which may be transmitted to humans following a bite from a rat – or possibly a mouse or certain other animals such as a weasel. Rarely, drinking unpasteurised milk contaminated with the causative bacteria has been responsible for cases of infection in people. The organisms involved are usually either *Streptobacillus moniliformis* or *Spirillum minus*. Cases are most prevalent in Japan but are also reported in North and South America, Africa and Europe. Symptoms include headache, fever, chills, malaise, vomiting, joint pains and skin rash. Treatment is by means of courses of antibiotics, such as penicillin or erythromycin, and bed rest along with good intake of fluids. Anyone bitten by a rat, including a laboratory rat, should always seek medical advice. People most at risk are those living in close proximity to wild rats in crowded and insanitary conditions.

Typhoid fever

Typhoid fever is a severe, gastrointestinal bacterial infection caused by *Salmonella typhi*. The infection is acquired by swallowing contaminated food or water and, although now rare in developed countries, typhoid is prevalent in many poorer parts of the world and people are particularly vulnerable when they are forced to live in crowded, insanitary conditions. Where standards of sanitation and sewage disposal are poor or nonexistent, water readily becomes contaminated while food may acquire the bacteria directly from an infected person or from someone who is a carrier. In countries where typhoid is prevalent, raw foods such as salads should be avoided and only sterile water should be drunk. Bottled or sterilised water should also be used for cleaning teeth. Any person suspected to be a carrier should not handle food and should receive treatment to eliminate the organism. Carriers do not always show signs of illness and in others an attack may only be mild and may not be diagnosed correctly, posing a risk to others.

Early symptoms include headache, malaise, nosebleeds, joint pain, sore throat, abdominal aches and tenderness. If not treated at this stage, there is a rise in temperature in a characteristic step-like pattern known as 'step-ladder' temperature rise. Changes in the appearance of the tongue, blood-streaked diarrhoea and a characteristic pink rash of 'rose spots' on the abdomen and (in some cases) the chest, are likely to be present. When the fever is at its height, the patient is too weak to rise and their heartbeat rate may slow down. There can be enlargement of the spleen, disturbance of liver function, anaemia, blood changes and loss of protein in the urine (proteinuria). Usually the symptoms gradually subside but, in severe cases, there may be ulceration of the intestinal wall and a risk of severe haemorrhage and/or peritonitis. Other complications include pneumonia, acute hepatitis, cholecystitis, meningitis, abscesses, endocarditis (inflammation of the membranes of the heart) and inflammation of the kidneys. The complications of typhoid fever can be fatal.

Treatment is by means of antibiotics and, in severe cases, hospital admission is needed so that these can be given intravenously. Intravenous fluids and electrolytes may also be required. Antibiotics used include chloramphenicol, ampicillin, ceftriaxone and cefoperazone. Scrupulous attention to hygiene is required and the patient should be isolated to prevent the infection from spreading. Clothing and bedding may need to be boiled or otherwise sterilised. A good recovery usually occurs with prompt treatment and in the absence of complications arising. The person needs to rest in bed until symptoms subside but complete recovery may take some considerable time. Follow-up tests are needed to ensure that the bacteria are no longer present and that the patient is not a carrier of the disease.

A preventative vaccine is available and this confers temporary protection against typhoid. Anyone travelling to a country where typhoid occurs should be vaccinated before departure.

Typhus

Typhus is a collective name for a group of febrile (feverish) bacterial infections caused by the *Rickettsiae* species of bacteria. Typhus is prevalent in many parts of the world and occurs in two forms, *endemic* and *epidemic*. The disease is transmitted to man via the bite of one of several species of external parasite, commonly the body louse. When the insect bites, the site becomes intensely itchy and, when scratched, the bacteria gain access to the blood circulation enabling the infection to occur. Epidemics of typhus often follow in the wake of war and natural disaster when weakened survivors are crowded together in insanitary conditions. Endemic typhus is a milder form of the infection. *R. prowazekii* is often responsible for the epidemic form and *R. typhi* for the endemic form. Other types include *murine typhus* (transmitted via rat or cat fleas, *R. felis*), *sylvatic typhus* (transmitted via bites from fleas that normally occur on flying squirrels) and Brill-Znesser disease (*recrudescent typhus*).

Epidemic typhus produces symptoms that include a severe headache, very high temperature and a skin rash that typically arises after 4 to 5 days. Also, there may be sensitivity to light (photophobia), wheezing and a cough, pains in the abdomen, nausea, ringing in the ears (tinnitus), deafness and delirium. Less commonly, mental effects, fits, and enlargement of the spleen, liver and lymph nodes may occur. Murine typhus produces similar symptoms and, rarely, confusion and hallucinations with a risk of kidney or liver failure or neurological disorders. Treatment is by means of antibiotics, especially doxycycline, tetracycline and chloramphenicol, and these must be continued for 2 days after symptoms subside. Recovery is normally complete in patients in whom severe complications involving major organs are absent but the infection carries a risk of mortality among vulnerable groups such as the very old, the young and those who are already ill. Preventative measures include not entering overcrowded areas, wearing close-fitting long clothes that cover the skin and taking weekly doses of doxycycline. A vaccine is available against *R. prowazekii* and this offers some protection.

Mediterranean spotted fever (MSF), boutonneuse fever

MSF, or boutonneuse fever, is a bacterial infection caused by a rickettsial organism, namely *Rickettsia conorii* and it is found in a species of tick, *Rhipicephalus sanguineus*, that is a common external parasite of dogs in several Mediterranean countries, including France, Spain, Portugal, Turkey, Greece and Italy. It is also found in areas around the Black Sea and in parts of India and Africa. Dogs can be affected by the illness and humans normally contract the infection incidentally through close contact with pets and ticks. Native dogs in endemic MSF areas often do not show clinical signs and usually have built up immunity through previous exposure. However, dogs from elsewhere, accompanying their owners on holiday, frequently show signs of illness but are immune following recovery. Cases are increasingly being reported among tourists visiting countries where the infection occurs.

Symptoms include headaches, fever, skin sores and eruptions, muscle pains, weight loss and diarrhoea. Liver and kidney function can be affected and there is a risk of liver or kidney failure. More commonly, there is a complete recovery following treatment with antibiotics and these include doxycycline, chloramphenicol, tetracycline and enrofloxacin. Travellers are advised to avoid being bitten by a tick and especially not to pet dogs in areas where the infection is known to occur. If a tick is picked up, it should be removed as quickly as possible and medical advice sought in the event of illness.

Ehrlichiosis, ehrlichia infection

Human ehrlichiosis, or ehrlichia infection, is a bacterial infection caused by various rickettsial species belonging to the genus *Ehrlichia*. The organisms are transmitted to humans via the bite of infected ticks that are normally parasitic on other mammals, especially dogs, horses, sheep, goats and cattle. Three types of *Ehrlichia* are known to cause human infections in the USA and a further one has been identified in Japan. Early symptoms include headache, fever, malaise, muscle aches and pains and sometimes, diarrhoea, vomiting, nausea, joint pains and confusion. A rash may occur, especially in children but rarely in adults. It is believed that some cases may remain undiagnosed if the illness is mild. Blood changes and alterations in liver enzymes are detected with laboratory analysis. There is a risk of serious complications in a small number of patients and those with weakened immunity are at greatest risk. Complications include prolonged fever, kidney failure, meningoencephalitis, fits, coma and adult respiratory distress syndrome and there is a risk of death in these instances. Treatment with antibiotics at an early stage normally produces a complete recovery and tetracycline or doxycycline are the antibiotics generally prescribed. Treatment is usually continued for 3 days after symptoms subside to ensure that all the infectious agents have been eliminated.

Rocky Mountain spotted fever

Rocky Mountain spotted fever is a serious, acute bacterial infection caused by a rickettsial organism called *Rickettsia rickettsii*. The bacteria are present in parasitic ticks that are found on many wild animals in the USA but this particular species does not occur in the UK or Europe. People acquire the illness following a bite from an infected tick (compare with **Lyme disease** on page 90).

Symptoms arise between 3 to 12 days after the tick bite and they include severe headache, high fever, nausea and vomiting, muscle stiffness and pain, chills and the appearance of a characteristic red rash that eventually spreads over much of the body. This may darken and ulcerate. The person may show signs of mental confusion, agitation, delirium, coma and death is possible.

A person showing early symptoms following a tick bite requires immediate medical treatment and this comprises a course of antibiotics such as tetracycline or chloramphenicol. The illness is normally curable if caught and treated promptly but may be fatal if treatment is delayed. A person who acquires a tick in an area where the disease is endemic should remove the insect as soon as possible and seek medical advice. Preventative measures include wearing protective clothing that covers all the skin and stout shoes or boots with thick socks. Also, the use of tick-repellent chemicals, such as diethyltoluamide (deet), to reduce the number of parasites is a further measure that may be employed.

Brucellosis, undulant fever, Malta fever, Mediterranean fever

Brucellosis, undulant fever, Malta fever, or Mediterranean fever, is a bacterial infection of animals that can also be readily passed to humans (a process called zoonosis). The causal organisms belong to the genus *Brucella* and there are many different species throughout the world inhabiting livestock and causing significant illness in infected animals and consequent economic losses. In animals, the principle effects of the disease are spontaneous abortion, lowered fertility, reduced production of milk and lameness. Three *Brucella* species commonly cause infection in humans and these are *B. melitensis* (found in sheep, goats and camels), *B. abortus* (found in cattle and camels) and *B. suis* (found in pigs). The disease is rare in humans in the UK and all reported cases in recent years have been acquired abroad. People can be infected by ingestion of contaminated products, particularly unpasteurised milk, cream or milk products such as soft cheeses and yoghurts. A further route of infection is by inhalation of particles following animal abortion, with farmers and veterinarians being at greater risk, or contaminated dust in abattoirs or laboratories. Finally, infection can occur through direct contact, with entry especially via the conjunctiva of the eyes and more rarely, through handling of live vaccines or from blood or bone marrow transplants.

Symptoms typically arise between 5 to 30 days following infection but in some instances this may be delayed for as long as 6 months. They can be vague and insidious in onset but usually there is a prolonged high temperature, headache, malaise, sweating, anorexia, weight loss, debility, pains in the joints and back, and often arthritis. There may be a dry cough and enlargement of the spleen and liver. The acute symptoms of the illness can last for many weeks and, although most people make a slow recovery, in some a chronic condition develops with relapses with severe arthritis, malaise and depression as frequent features. *B. melitensis* and *B. suis* generally produce a more severe human illness than *B. abortus* with abscesses being a feature of *B. suis* infection.

Treatment is by means of symptom relief and antibiotics, including tetracyclines, co-trimoxazole and gentamycin. Tetramycin and streptomycin are prescribed for the chronic form. Brucellosis is rarely fatal but there is a risk of death from serious complications such as meningitis or pneumonia. In developed countries, there is rigorous testing of cattle and the slaughter of infected animals to limit the risk to human health, and all dairy products are pasteurised. However, brucellosis is endemic in Portugal, Spain, Southern France, Italy, Greece, Turkey, North Africa, Eastern Europe, Asia, the Middle East, the Caribbean and Central and South America. A person visiting any of these countries should not consume unpasteurised dairy products.

Yellow fever

Yellow fever is an extremely serious viral infection caused by organisms belonging to the group *Flaviviridae*. Humans acquire the illness through being bitten by infected mosquitoes that belong to the genus *Aedes*, commonly *Aedes egyptii*. Yellow fever is endemic in 33 mainly impoverished countries located within Africa and South America and their combined populations of around 468 million people are at risk of catching the disease. Yellow fever is more properly a jungle disease in which the reservoir for the virus is monkeys (the 'sylvatic cycle').

Humans were initially infected through being bitten by mosquitoes in the jungle. A return of people to the urban environment has resulted in there being a reservoir of infection among humans, and the pattern is of a certain level of cases with periodic epidemics. A characteristic feature is hepatitis with jaundice and this produces a yellow colouration of the skin – hence yellow fever.

Symptoms appear in stages and vary greatly in severity with some people having none or only a very mild illness. The incubation period is between 3 to 16 days following a bite from an infected mosquito. In the acute illness, symptoms have a sudden onset and early, first stage ones include a very high fever, violent headache, vomiting, rise then fall in pulse rate, facial flushing, muscle pains, loss of fluid and irritability. The amount of urine passed decreases and protein is lost in the urine, indicating inflammation of the kidneys. However, in the majority of cases, the fever subsides in 3 to 4 days and the patient gradually recovers and feels better – the second stage. But around 25% of people experience a severe resumption of illness – the third stage – with hepatitis and development of jaundice, anaemia, kidney inflammation, vomiting blood and bleeding from the mouth, nose and mucous membranes. There is a low heartbeat and fever and possible kidney failure, delirium, fits, coma and death. Most patients who develop haemorrhages die within a short space of time. The overall mortality rate is between 5% and 40% with more deaths occurring during epidemics.

In mild cases, treatment consists of bed rest, drinking plenty of fluid and taking analgesics (although paracetamol should be avoided). Serious cases necessitate admittance to hospital for intensive supporting nursing care. Fluids and electrolytes are given intravenously along with measures to cool the patient and bring down fever. There are no effective medicines against the causal virus. A vaccine is available that confers protection after about 10 days following the injection. Anyone travelling to an affected area should ensure vaccination before departure and the injection needs to be repeated every 10 years. Use of insecticide repellents and protective clothing to cover exposed skin are measures that can be employed to try and avoid being bitten by mosquitoes.

Lassa fever

Lassa fever is a serious and highly contagious viral infection that is endemic in some African countries and was first identified in Lassa in Nigeria. Cases have been reported among Europeans who have visited countries where the disease occurs. The causal organism is an arenavirus that is harboured and spread by rats, being excreted in droppings and urine. People can be infected by touching contaminated surfaces or substances (the virus

may enter through a cut or the mouth), inhalation of infective particles or, more commonly, by eating contaminated food.
Person to person infection can occur via body waste, blood or
saliva. The incubation period is usually about 10 days but can be
shorter or longer in some cases.

Early symptoms include headache, fever, sore throat, cough,
chills, abdominal pains, muscle pains and lethargy. Later there
is vomiting, anorexia, weight loss and severe pains in the chest.
The sore throat worsens and there may be a yellowish-white
discharge and vomiting continues with severe abdominal pains.
There may be swelling of the neck, face and conjunctiva of the
eyes due to oedema, ringing in the ears, rash, internal bleeding
and effects on heartbeat and blood pressure. Death may follow
with mortality being particularly high among pregnant women or
in those who have just given birth.

There is no effective treatment against the virus. A person
who is ill with Lassa fever requires admittance to hospital for
intensive, supportive nursing care with correction of fluid and
electrolyte imbalance being particularly important. The patient
must be kept in isolation and barrier nursing methods employed.
Antiviral agents such as ribavirin have been tried with some
promising results. If travelling to a country where the disease
occurs, vigilance is needed with regard to food hygiene and it is
wise to avoid areas where rats may be present.

Dengue fever, 'breakbone fever', dandy fever

Dengue fever, or 'breakbone fever', or dandy fever, is a viral
infection transmitted to humans via the bite of an *Aedes* species
of mosquito, usually *Aedes egypti*. The causal organisms belong
to the genus *Flavivirus* and there are four species identified as
being involved. The illness is endemic in Africa, South America,
Southeast Asia, the Eastern Mediterranean and Western Pacific.
A more severe form, known as *dengue haemorrhagic fever*, is

responsible for around 24,000 deaths each year. The milder form of dengue produces initial flu-like symptoms, including headache, fever, aches and pains in muscles and joints, malaise and weakness. Some people go on to develop a rash and extreme fatigue before symptoms gradually subside. This form is the one that usually affects travellers to a dengue area. Most people with mild illness do not require treatment although fatigue can persist for 2 to 3 months.

In classic dengue, there is a sudden onset of a very high temperature, intense headache, severe joint and muscle pains (hence 'breakbone') and a characteristic bright red rash that appears first on the legs and chest but may spread to other areas. Abdominal pains, nausea and vomiting may also arise. Usually, the fever lasts for about a week and shows a biphasic pattern with a lowering of temperature after the initial peak, followed by a second lower peak. In dengue haemorrhagic fever, the symptoms are much more severe with a very high temperature, intense headache, internal bleeding, blood changes, enlarged liver and in some instances, circulatory fever and collapse. If death occurs it is usually caused by these effects on the circulation collectively called dengue shock syndrome (DSS). Treatment in severe cases is by means of supportive therapy that includes giving fluids and electrolytes intravenously and possibly, a transfusion of blood platelets. There is no preventative vaccine and protection comprises avoidance of being bitten by mosquitoes by wearing clothing that covers the skin and using insect repellent lotions. The aedes mosquitoes are active only by day.

West Nile virus (WNV)

West Nile virus is a mosquito-borne infection in which the causal organisms are flaviviruses. The disease was first identified in Uganda but it is now endemic in many parts of the world, including Africa, West Asia, the Middle East and North America. Many species of mosquito have been identified as insect vectors but most commonly, those belonging to the genus *Culex*, particularly *Culex pipiens*, *C. salinanu* and *C. restuans*. The disease is mild in most people and it usually causes few or no symptoms (80% of cases). When symptoms do occur, they typically arise after an incubation period of 1 to 6 days and produce a mild, flu-like illness with headache, fever, muscle pains and a rash. About 1 in every 150 people develop much more serious neurological symptoms, meningitis or encephalitis. In these patients, a severe headache, stiff neck, mental confusion, fits, paralysis and coma may all arise and fatality rates can be as high as 30%, especially in those aged over 50 years or those who are already suffering from some other illness or disorder. Treatment is supportive and in severe cases, intensive nursing in hospital is required. There is no vaccine available and prevention takes the form of avoidance of mosquito bites by using cover-all clothing and insect repellent lotions.

SARS (Severe acute respiratory syndrome)

SARS is a severe respiratory viral disease that was first identified in 2002. Between November 2002 and July 2003, an outbreak of SARS in southern China caused an eventual 8,273 cases and 775 deaths worldwide. It is believed to have spread to other continents through international travel. The causative agent has been identified as a coronavirus, although it is possible other infectious agents are associated with some cases. The incubation period is about 10 days and symptoms are those of severe flu, including fever, headache, sore throat, cough, chills, aches and pains and malaise. In about 4% of people, complications develop in the form of pneumonia and this can prove fatal, especially amongst the young and elderly. It is thought that the virus is transmitted by the airborne inhalation of infective particles via coughing and sneezing. There is no treatment other than supportive care, and patients must be isolated in hospital and nursed using barrier methods.

Chapter 12

WHEN TO SEEK MEDICAL HELP

The general advice that applies to all conditions is that if you have a symptom that is worrying you and especially if it has been present for more than 3 weeks then you should obtain medical help. However, there are certain criteria attached to the occurrence of headache that should prompt a doctor being called without delay. These are:

- A first intense headache occurring over the age of 50 years.
- An intense headache that comes on very suddenly.
- An intense headache after exertion.
- An intense headache with fever and/or rash or vomiting.
- A headache with drowsiness, difficulty in waking, vision disturbance, loss of coordination or balance.
- A change in the usual character of migraines.
- Aura symptoms that are always on the same side or persist for more than an hour.
- Aura symptoms without headache.

Part Two

COMPLEMENTARY THERAPIES AND HOW THEY CAN HELP

Chapter 13

MIND AND BODY

When we are completely overwhelmed by our emotions, we become the sum total of our thoughts, rather than the instigator and controller of them. To stop this, the mind must be stilled, all thoughts put on hold. To rediscover that our thoughts are under our control is incredibly liberating and empowering. Taking control enables us to see things as they really are, without being hindered by associative thoughts, and allows us to respond more appropriately, because our response is direct, based on the here and now. For example, meditation, a complementary therapy, helps us to live in the here and now, and to see ourselves as the controller of our own mind and thoughts. In so doing, it also helps us to have a deeper understanding of what is happening to us including any pain we may be experiencing.

Ever since the French philosopher, Rene Descartes, uttered 'I think therefore I am', we have been encouraged to identify ourselves with our conscious minds. Descartes' philosophy of 'dualism' prompted us to view our minds as distinct from our bodies: the former was an organ of reason and imagination, the latter an engine.

This did not happen to the same extent in the East, where a more holistic, integrated approach to the human mind and body was observed, as in acupressure and acupuncture, which relate to the emotions as well as physical pressure points.

In the West, however, medicine approached the body rather as mechanics approached the car. The symptoms of physical ailments were treated with little reference to what circumstances caused them to manifest themselves. Who would worry about how a car's tyre became punctured? Even worse perhaps, the human body was regarded as a series of separate parts, each to be treated by a different specialist, with little reference to the rest of the body.

This specialist approach has led to enormous medical and surgical achievements. Many diseases have been virtually obliterated due to vaccines, diseased organs need no longer threaten life if a donor can be found, and even in the field of mental illness drugs have been developed that can suppress some of the distressing symptoms of conditions such as schizophrenia and manic depression. The rub is that Western medicine, so advanced in many other ways, seems to have drawn a veil over the link between psyche and health.

Holistic (from the Greek *holos*, meaning 'whole'), alternative medicine has become increasingly popular in the West, especially amongst people who feel that the use of drugs can only help to a certain extent. The holistic approach regards the body and mind as one, where everything is connected to everything else, and nothing can happen to one part without everything else being affected.

Rather than prescribe drugs, a doctor who believes in the holistic approach to medicine and who understands the value of complementary medicine may prescribe an alternative way of nudging the body back into gear. Furthermore, and perhaps most importantly, the patient is expected to participate in the healing process. Pharmacology has accustomed us to the idea that the patient's role is a passive one: we expect the doctor to do all the work, from diagnosis to selecting the right chemical. Holistic medicine is more honest in that it acknowledges it can only help to stimulate the body into healing itself, which in fact it is usually very capable of doing, given the right circumstances. There is indeed a role for complementary therapies in the treatment, management and prevention of headaches and migraines, and in the following chapters we explore (in alphabetical order) some of the complementary therapies that may have something to offer anyone who has suffered the pain and discomfort of a headache.

Chapter 14

ACUPRESSURE

Origins

This is an ancient form of healing combining massage and acupuncture, practised over 3,000 years ago in Japan and China. It was developed into its current form using a system of special massage points and is today still practised widely in the Japanese home environment.

Certain 'pressure points' are located in various parts of the body and these are used by the practitioner through massaging firmly with the thumb or fingertip. These points are the same as those utilised in acupuncture. There are various ways of working and the pressure can be applied by the practitioner's fingers, thumbs, knees, palms of the hand, etc. Relief from pain can be quite rapid at times, depending upon its cause, while other more persistent problems can take longer to improve.

Acupressure is said to enhance the body's own method of healing, thereby preventing illness and improving energy levels. The pressure exerted is believed to regulate the energy that flows along the meridians – the pathways or energy channels, believed to be related to the internal organs that run along the length of the body. Most of these 14 meridians are named after the organs of the body, such as the liver and stomach, but there are four exceptions which are called the 'pericardium', 'triple heater', 'conception' and 'governor'. Specifically named meridian lines may also be used to treat ailments other than those relating to it.

Treatment

Ailments claimed to have been treated successfully are migraine and circulatory problems, back pain, asthma, digestive problems, and insomnia, amongst others. Changes in diet, regular exercise and certain self-checking methods may also be recommended by your practitioner. It must be borne in mind that some painful symptoms are the onset of serious illness so you should always first consult your GP.

Before any treatment commences, a patient will be asked for details of his (or her) lifestyle and diet, and their pulse rate will be taken along with any relevant past history relating to the current problem. The person will be requested to lie on a mattress on the floor or on a firm table, and comfortable but loose-fitting clothing is best so that the practitioner can work most effectively on the energy channels. No oils are used on the body and there is no equipment. Each session lasts from approximately half an hour to an hour. Once the pressure is applied, and this can be done in a variety of ways particular to each practitioner, varying sensations may be felt. Some points may feel sore or tender and there may be some discomfort such as a deep pain or coolness. However, it is believed that this form of massage works quickly so that any tenderness soon passes. The number of treatments will vary from patient to patient, according to how the person responds and what problem or ailment is being treated. Weekly visits may be needed if a specific disorder is being treated while other people may go whenever they feel in need. It is advisable for women who are pregnant to check with their practitioner first since some of the acupressure methods are not recommended during pregnancy.

Acupressure can be practised safely at home although it is usually better for one person to perform the massage on another. Common problems, such as headache, constipation and toothache, can be treated quite simply, although, if the pressure points are over stimulated, there is the possibility of a problem worsening first before an improvement occurs. You should, however, see your doctor if any ailment persists. To treat headache, facial soreness, toothache and menstrual pain, locate the fleshy piece of skin between the thumb and forefinger and squeeze firmly, pressing towards the forefinger. The pressure should be applied for about 5 minutes and either hand can be used. This point is known as 'large intestine 4'.

To aid digestive problems in both adults and babies, for example to settle infantile colic, the point known as 'stomach 36' is utilised, which is located on the outer side of the leg about 75 mm (3 ins) down from the knee. This point should be quite simple to find as it can often feel slightly tender. It should be pressed quite firmly and strongly for about 5 to 10 minutes with the thumb.

When practising acupressure massage on someone else and before treatment begins, ensure that the person is warm, relaxed, comfortable and wearing loose-fitting clothing and that he (or she) is lying on a firm mattress or rug on the floor. To discover the areas that need to be worked on, press firmly over the body and see which areas are tender. These tender areas on the body correspond to an organ that is not working correctly. To commence massage using fingertips or thumbs, a pressure of about 4.5 kg (10 lbs) should be exerted. The massage movements should be performed very quickly, about 50 to 100 times every minute, and some discomfort is likely (which will soon pass) but there should be no pain. Particular care should be taken to avoid causing pain on the face, stomach or over any joints. If a baby or young child is being massaged, then considerably less pressure should be used. If there is any doubt as to the correct amount, exert a downwards pressure on bathroom scales to ascertain the weight being used. There is no need to hurry from one point to another since approximately 5 to 15 minutes is needed at each point for adults (but only about 30 seconds for babies or young children).

It is possible that as many as 20 sessions may be necessary for persistent conditions causing pain, with greater intervals of time between treatments as matters improve. It is not advisable to try anything that is at all complicated, or to treat an illness such as arthritis, and a trained practitioner will obviously be able to provide the best level of treatment and help. To get in touch with a reputable practitioner who has completed the relevant training, contact the appropriate professional body.

Chapter 15

ACUPUNCTURE

Origins

Acupuncture is an ancient Chinese therapy that involves inserting needles into the skin at specific points of the body. The word 'acupuncture' originated from a Dutch physician, William Ten Rhyne, who had been living in Japan during the latter part of the seventeenth century and it was he who introduced it to Europe. The term means literally 'prick with a needle'. The earliest textbook on acupuncture, dating from approximately 400 BC, was called *Nei Ching Su Wen*, which means 'Yellow Emperor's Classic of Internal Medicine'. Also recorded at about the same time was the successful saving of a patient's life by acupuncture, the person having been expected to die whilst in a coma. Legend has it that acupuncture was developed when it was realised that soldiers who recovered from arrow wounds were sometimes also healed of other diseases from which they were suffering. Acupuncture was very popular with British doctors in the early 1800s for pain relief and to treat fever. There was also a specific article on the successful treatment of rheumatism that appeared in *The Lancet*. Until the end of the Ching dynasty in China in

1911, acupuncture was slowly developed and improved, but then medicine from the West increased in popularity. However, more recently there has been a revival of interest in acupuncture and it is again widely practised throughout China. Also, nowadays the use of laser beams and electrical currents is found to give an increased stimulative effect when using acupuncture needles.

The specific points of the body into which acupuncture needles are inserted are located along meridians. These are the pathways or energy channels of the body and are believed to be related to the internal organs. This energy is known as *qi* and the needles are used to decrease or increase the flow of energy, or to unblock it if it is impeded. Traditional Chinese medicine sees the body as being comprised of two natural forces known as the *yin* and *yang*. These two forces are complementary to each other but also opposing. The yin is the female force and is calm and passive, representing the dark, cold, swelling and moisture. The yang is the male force and it is stimulating and aggressive, representing the heat and light, contraction and dryness. It is believed that the cause of ailments and diseases is due to an imbalance of these forces in the body, e.g. if a person is suffering from a headache or hypertension then this is because of an excess of yang. If, however, there is an excess of yin, this might result in tiredness, feeling cold and fluid retention.

The aim of acupuncture is to establish whether there is an imbalance of yin and yang and to rectify it by using the needles at certain points on the body. Traditionally there were 365 points but more have been found in the intervening period and nowadays there can be as many as 2,000. There are 14 meridians and 12 of these are called after the organs they represent, including the lung, kidney, heart and stomach, as well as the triple heater or warmer, which relates to the activity of the endocrine glands and the control of temperature, and the pericardium which is concerned with seasonal activity and also regulates the circulation of the blood. The remaining 2 meridians both run straight up the body's midline: the *du* meridian, or governor vessel, and the ren meridian, or conception vessel. The du is much shorter, extending from the head down to the mouth, while the ren starts at the chin and extends to the base of the trunk. There are several factors that can change the flow of qi (also known as *shi* or *ch'i*), and they can be of an emotional, physical or environmental nature. The flow may have changed to become too slow or fast or been diverted or blocked so that the incorrect organ is involved, and the acupuncturist has to ensure that the flow returns to normal.

There are many painful afflictions for which acupuncture can be used. Ailments which respond well to acupuncture include neck, shoulder and back pain and osteoarthritis in the knee, and recent research has indicated that acupuncture is an effective treatment for all types of headaches and migraine. Acupuncture has also been successfully used to alleviate other disorders such as stress, allergy, colitis, digestive troubles, insomnia, asthma, etc. It has been claimed that withdrawal symptoms (experienced by people who are trying to stop smoking and other forms of addiction) have been helped as well.

Qualified acupuncturists complete a three-year training course. They also need qualifications in the related disciplines of anatomy, pathology, physiology and diagnosis before they can belong to a professional association. It is very important that a fully qualified acupuncturist, who is a member of the relevant professional body, is consulted because at the present time, any unqualified person can use the title 'acupuncturist'.

Treatment

At a consultation, the traditional acupuncturist uses a set method of ancient rules to determine the acupuncture points. The texture and colouring of the skin, type of skin, posture and movement and the tongue will all be examined and noted, as will the patient's voice. These different factors are all needed for the Chinese diagnosis. A number of questions will be asked concerning the diet, amount of exercise taken, lifestyle, fears and phobias, sleeping patterns and reactions to stress. If, for example, the patient is suffering from headaches, he (or she) will be asked specific questions about their headaches. Each wrist has 6 pulses, and each of these stand for a main organ and its function. The pulses are felt (known as palpating), and by this means acupuncturists are able to diagnose any problems relating to the flow of qi and if there is any disease present in the internal organs. The first consultation may last an hour, especially if detailed questioning is necessary along with the palpation.

The needles used in acupuncture are disposable and made of a very fine stainless steel and come already sealed in a sterile pack. They can be sterilised by the acupuncturist in a machine known as an autoclave but simply using boiling water is not adequate for this purpose. (Diseases such as HIV and hepatitis can be passed on by using unsterilised needles.) Acupuncture points to treat headaches are located all over the body and needles may be placed, for example, along the legs, arms, and shoulders. Once the needle is inserted into the skin it is twisted between the acupuncturist's thumb and forefinger to spread or draw the energy from a point. The depth to which the needle is inserted can vary from just below the skin to up to 12 mm (half an inch) and different sensations may be felt, such as a tingling around the area of insertion or a loss of sensation at that point. Up to 15 needles can be inserted and the time they are left in for varies from a few minutes to half an hour and this is dependent on a number of factors such as how the patient has reacted to previous treatment and the ailment from which he (or she) is suffering.

Patients can generally expect to feel an improvement after 4 to 6 sessions of therapy, the beneficial effects occurring gradually, particularly if the ailment has obvious and long-standing symptoms. Other diseases such as asthma will probably take longer before any definite improvement is felt. It is possible that some patients may not feel any improvement at all, or even feel worse after the first session and this is probably due to the energies in the body being overstimulated. To correct this, the acupuncturist will gradually use fewer needles and for a shorter period of time. If no improvement is felt after about 6 to 8 treatments, then it is doubtful whether acupuncture will be of any help. For general body maintenance and health, most traditional acupuncturists suggest that sessions be arranged at the time of seasonal changes.

How does it work?

There has been a great deal of research, particularly by the Chinese, who have produced many books detailing a high success rate for acupuncture in treating a variety of disorders. These results are, however, viewed cautiously in the West as methods of conducting clinical trials vary from East to West. Nevertheless trials have been carried out in the West and it has been discovered that a pain message can be stopped from reaching the brain using acupuncture. The signal would normally travel along a nerve but it is possible to 'close a gate' on the nerve, thereby preventing the message from reaching the brain, hence preventing the perception of pain. Acupuncture is believed to work by blocking the pain signal. However, doctors stress that pain can be a warning of something wrong or of the occurrence of a particular disease, such as cancer, which requires an orthodox remedy or method of treatment.

It has also been discovered that there are substances produced by the body that are connected with pain relief. These substances are called endorphins and encephalins, and they are natural opiates. Studies from all over the world show that acupuncture stimulates the release of these opiates into the central nervous system, thereby giving pain relief. The amount of opiates released has a direct bearing on the degree of pain relief. Acupuncture is a widely used form of anaesthesia in China where, for suitable patients, it is said to be extremely effective (90%). It is used successfully during childbirth, dentistry and for operations.

Orthodox doctors in the West now accept that heat treatment, massage and needles used on a sensitive part of the skin afford relief from pain caused by disease elsewhere. These areas are known as trigger points, and they are not always situated close to the organ that is affected by disease. It has been found that approximately three-quarters of these trigger points are the same as the points used in Chinese acupuncture. Recent research has also shown that it is possible to find the acupuncture points by the use of electronic instruments as they register less electrical resistance than other areas of skin. As yet, no evidence has been found to substantiate the existence of meridians.

Chapter 16

THE ALEXANDER TECHNIQUE

Origins

The Alexander technique is a practical and simple method of learning to focus attention on how we use ourselves during daily activities. Frederick Mathias Alexander (1869–1955), an Australian therapist, demonstrated that the difficulties many people experience in learning, in control of performance, and in physical functioning are caused by unconscious habits. These habits interfere with your natural poise and your capacity to learn. When you stop interfering with the innate coordination of the body, you can take on more complex activities with greater self-confidence and presence of mind. It is about learning to bring into our conscious awareness the choices we make, as we make them. Gentle hands-on and verbal instruction reveal the underlying principles of human coordination, allow the student to experience and observe their own habitual patterns, and give the means for release and change.

The Alexander technique is based on correct posture so that the body is able to function naturally and with the minimum amount of muscular effort. F. M. Alexander was also an actor and found that he was losing his voice when performing but after rest his condition temporarily improved. Although he received medical help, the condition was not cured and it occurred to him that whilst acting he might be doing something that caused the problem. To see what this might be he performed his act in front of a mirror and saw what happened when he was about to speak. He experienced difficulty in breathing and lowered his head, thus making himself shorter. He realised that the strain of remembering his lines and having to project his voice so that people furthest away in the audience would be able to hear, was causing him a great deal of stress and the way he reacted was a quite natural reflex action. In fact, even thinking about having to project his voice made the symptoms recur and from this he concluded that there must be a close connection between body and mind. He was determined to try and improve the situation and gradually, by watching and altering his stance and posture and his mental attitude to his performance on stage, matters improved. He was able to act and speak on stage and use his body in a more relaxed and natural fashion.

In 1904 Alexander travelled to London where he had decided to let others know about his method of retraining the body. He soon became very popular with other actors who appreciated the benefits of using his technique. Other public figures, including Aldous Huxley, the author, also benefited. Later he went to America, achieving considerable success and international recognition for his technique. At the age of 78 he suffered a stroke but by using his method he managed to regain the use of all his faculties – an achievement that amazed his doctors.

Armouring

Most of us are unconsciously armouring ourselves in relation to our environment. This is hard work and often leaves us feeling anxious, alienated, depressed and unlovable. Armouring is a deeply unconscious behaviour that has probably gone on since early childhood, maybe even since infancy. Yet it is a habit we can unlearn in the present through careful self-observation. We can unlearn our use of excess tension in our thoughts, movements, and relationships.

Treatment

The Alexander technique is said to be completely harmless, encouraging an agreeable state between mind and body. It is also helpful for a number of disorders such as headaches and back pain.

Today, Alexander training schools can be found all over the world. A simple test to determine if people can benefit is to observe their posture. People frequently do not even stand correctly and this can encourage aches and pains if the body is unbalanced. It is incorrect to stand with round shoulders or to slouch. This often looks uncomfortable and discomfort may be felt. Sometimes people will hold themselves too erect and unbending, which again can have a bad effect. The correct posture and balance for the body needs the least muscular effort but the body will be aligned correctly. When walking one should not slouch, hold the head down or have the shoulders stooped. The head should be balanced correctly above the spine with the shoulders relaxed. It is suggested that the weight of the body should be felt being transferred from one foot to the other whilst walking.

Once a teacher has been consulted, all movements and how the body is used will be observed. Many muscles are used in everyday activities, and over the years bad habits can develop unconsciously, with stress also affecting the use of muscles. This can be demonstrated in people gripping a pen with too much force or holding the steering wheel of a car too tightly whilst driving. Muscular tension can be a serious problem affecting some people often leading to tension head-aches. When the head, neck and back are forced out of line, this can lead to rounded shoulders with the head held forward and the back curved. If this situation is not altered and the body is not re-aligned correctly, the spine will become curved with a hump possibly developing. This leads to back pain and puts a strain on internal organs such as the chest and lungs.

An Alexander teacher guides a person, as he (or she) moves, to use less tension. The instructor works by monitoring the student's posture and reminding him or her to implement tiny changes in movement to eradicate the habit of excess tension. Students learn to stop bracing themselves up, or to stop collaps-ing into themselves. As awareness grows, it becomes easier to recognise and relinquish the habit of armouring and dissolve the artificial barriers we put between ourselves and others.

An analogy of this process can be seen in the now famil-iar three-dimensional Magic Eye Art. With our ordinary way of looking we see only a mass of dots. When we shift to the 'Magic Eye' way of seeing, a three-dimensional object appears. Through the Alexander technique a similar type of experience is available. But the three-dimensional object we experience is ourselves.

No force is used by the teacher other than some gentle manipulation to start pupils off correctly. Some teachers use light pushing methods on the back and hips, etc, while others might first ensure that the pupil is relaxed and then pull gently on the neck, which stretches the body. Any bad postures will be corrected by the teacher and the pupil will be shown how best to alter this so that muscles will be used most effectively and with the least effort. Any manipulation that is used will be to ease the body into a more relaxed and natural position. It is helpful to be completely aware of using the technique not only on the body but also with the mind. With frequent use of the Alexander technique for posture and the release of tension, the muscles and the body should be used correctly with a consequent improvement in, for example, the manner of walking and sitting and a significant lessening of tension headaches.

The length of time for each lesson can vary from about 30 minutes to 45 minutes and the number of lessons is usually between 10 and 30, by which time pupils should have gained sufficient knowledge to continue practising the technique by themselves. Once a person has learned how to improve their posture, he (or she) carries the body in a more upright manner. The technique has been found to be of benefit to dancers, athletes and those having to speak in public. Other disorders claimed to have been treated successfully are headaches caused by tension, depressive states, anxiety, asthma, hypertension, respiratory problems, colitis, osteoarthritis and rheumatoid arthritis, sciatica and peptic ulcer. The Alexander technique is recommended for all ages and types of people as their overall quality of life, both mental and physical, can be improved. People can learn how to resist stress and one eminent professor experienced a great improvement in a variety of ways: in quality of sleep; lessening of high blood pressure and improved mental awareness. He even found that his ability to play a musical instrument had improved.

The Alexander technique can be applied to two positions adopted every day, namely sitting in a chair and sitting at a desk.

To be seated in the correct manner the head should be comfortably balanced, with no tension in the shoulders, and a small gap between the knees (if the legs are crossed the spine and pelvis become out of line or twisted) and the soles of the feet should be flat on the floor. It is incorrect to sit with the head lowered and the shoulders slumped forward because the stomach becomes restricted and breathing may also be affected. On the other hand, it is also incorrect to hold the body in a stiff and erect position.

To sit correctly while working at a table or a desk, the body should be held upright but in a relaxed manner with any bending movement coming from the hips and with the seat flat on the chair. If writing, the pen should be held lightly and if using a computer one should ensure that the arms are relaxed and feel comfortable. The chair should be set at a comfortable height with regard to the level of the desk. There has been some scientific research carried out that concurs with the beliefs that Alexander formed, such as the relationship between mind and body (the thought of doing an action actually triggering a physical reaction or tension). Today, doctors do not have any opposition to the Alexander technique and may recommend it on occasions.

Although the Alexander technique does not treat specific symptoms, you can encourage a marked improvement in your overall health, alertness, and performance by consciously eliminating harmful habits that cause physical and emotional stress, including tension headaches, and by becoming more aware of how you engage in your activities.

Chapter 17

AROMATHERAPY

Healing through aromatherapy

Aromatherapy is a method of healing using very concentrated essential oils that are often highly aromatic and are extracted from plants. Constituents of the oils confer the characteristic perfume or odour given off by a particular plant. Essential oils help the plant in some way to complete its cycle of growth and reproduction. For example, some oils may attract insects for the purpose of pollination; others may render it distasteful as a source of food. Any part of a plant – the stems, leaves, flowers, fruits, seeds, roots or bark – may produce essential oils or essences but often only in minute amounts. Different parts of the same plant may produce their own form of oil. An example of this is the orange, which produces oils with different properties in the flowers, fruits and leaves.

Origins

Art and writings from the ancient civilisations of Egypt, China and Persia show that plant essences were used and valued by priests, physicians and healers. Plant essences have been used throughout the ages for healing, in incense for religious rituals, in perfumes and embalming ointments, and for culinary purposes. There are many Biblical references that give an insight into the uses of plant oils and the high value that was attached to them. Throughout the course of human history the healing properties of plants and their essential oils has been recognised and most people probably had some knowledge about their use. It was only in more recent times, with the great developments in science and orthodox medicine, particularly the manufacture of antibiotics and synthetic drugs, that knowledge and interest in the older methods of healing declined. However, in the last few years there has been a great rekindling of interest in the practice of aromatherapy with many people turning to this form of treatment.

Essential oils

Extraction of essential oils – steam distillation, solvent extraction, maceration, defleurage, enfleurage

Since any part of a plant may produce essential oils, the method of extraction depends upon the site and accessibility of the essence in each particular case. The oils are produced by special minute cells or glands and are released naturally by the plant in small amounts over a prolonged period of time when needed. In order to harvest the oils in appreciable amounts, it is usually necessary to collect a large quantity of the part of the plant needed and to subject the material to a process that causes the oil glands to burst.

One of the most common methods is *steam distillation*. The plant material is placed tightly into a press or still and steamed at a high temperature. This causes the oil glands to burst and the essential oil vaporises into the steam. This is then cooled to separate the oil from the water. Sometimes water is used for distillation rather than steam.

Another method involves dissolving the plant material in a solvent or alcohol and is called *solvent extraction*. This involves placing the material in a centrifuge, which rotates at high speed, and then extracting the essential oils by means of a low temperature distillation process. Substances obtained in this way may be called resins or absolutes.

A further method is called *maceration* in which the plant is soaked in hot oil. The plant cells collapse and release their essential oils, and the whole mixture is then separated and purified by a process called *defleurage*. If fat is used instead of oil, the process is called *enfleurage*. These methods produce a purer oil that is usually more expensive than one obtained by distillation. The essential oils used in aromatherapy tend to be costly as vast quantities of plant material are required to produce them and the methods used to obtain them are complex and costly.

Storage and use of essential oils

Essential oils are highly concentrated, volatile and aromatic. They readily evaporate and change and deteriorate if exposed to light, heat and air. Hence pure oils need to be stored carefully in brown glass bottles at a moderate temperature away from direct light. They can be stored for 1 or 2 years in this way. For most purposes in aromatherapy, essential oils are used in a dilute form, being added either to water or to another oil, called the base or carrier oil. The base oil is often a vegetable oil, such as olive or safflower, both of which have nutrient and beneficial properties. An essential/carrier oil mixture has a short useful life of 2 or 3 months, so they are usually mixed at the time of use and in small amounts.

Base oils

Because essential oils are extremely concentrated and also because of their tendency to evaporate rapidly, they need to be diluted with carrier or base oils. Generally it is not advised that essential oils should be applied undiluted to the skin, although there are one or two specific exceptions. It is very important to use a high quality base oil. For example, oils such as baby or mineral oil have very poor penetrating qualities which will hamper the passage of the essential oil through the skin. Indeed, it would be better to use a good quality vegetable or nut oil for babies in preference to proprietary baby oils as the vegetable oil is more easily absorbed and contains more nutrients.

Although the choice of base oil is largely a matter of personal preference, it is useful to note that many vegetable oils possess therapeutic properties of their own. Sweet almond, soya bean, sunflower, jojoba, olive, grapeseed, hazelnut, avocado, corn or safflower will all provide a suitable base for essential oils, although these should preferably be of the cold-pressed variety with higher nutrient levels.

Pure essential oils should retain their potency for 1 to 2 years, but once diluted in a base oil they will only last for 3 months or so before spoiling. They should also be stored at a fairly constant room temperature in corked dark glass bottles or flip-top containers as they will deteriorate quickly when subjected to extremes of light and temperature. Adding some vitamin E or wheatgerm oil to the mixture can help prolong its usefulness. For massage oils, it is best to make up a very small quantity of essential oil in base oil for each application because of its poor aromatherapy keeping qualities.

Below is a very rough guide to the dilution of essential oils. However, you will find many variations and differing opinions on this depending on the preference of individual therapists, and their recipes will differ accordingly. Be aware that some oils can be toxic if they are not correctly diluted.

Base oil	Essential oil
100ml	20–60 drops
25ml	7–25 drops
1 teaspoon (5 ml)	3–5 drops

Blending essential oils

Essences can be blended to treat specific ailments, and some aromatherapy books contain precise recipes for blends. When two or more essential oils are working together in harmony, this is known as a 'synergistic' blend. Obviously, it takes many years of experience to know which combinations of plant essences will work most effectively together, but as a rough guide, oils extracted from plants of the same botanical family will usually blend and work well together, However, it is by no means necessary to stick rigidly to this rule as other combinations may be just as successful. Also, a number of other factors need to be taken into account when preparing a blend of oils for a patient, such as the nature of his (or her) complaint and their personality or frame of mind. For home use, it is not usually beneficial to blend more than 3 oils for any one preparation.

How essential oils work

Inhalation, application and bathing are the three main methods used to encourage the entry of essential oils into the body. When inhaled, the extremely volatile oils may enter via the olfactory system, and permeation of the skin occurs when they are diluted and applied externally. By bathing in essential oils, we can inhale and absorb the oils through the skin simultaneously.

Little is known about how essential oils actually affect the mind and the body, although research is currently ongoing in the USA and the UK. However, the effectiveness of aromatherapy has been supported by recent research in central Europe, the USA, the UK and Australia. It appears that most essential oils are antiseptic and bactericidal to some degree, whilst some even seem to be effective in fighting viral infections.

On inhalation, essential oil molecules are received by receptor cells in the lining of the nose, which will transmit signals to the brain. Electrochemical messages received by the olfactory centre in the brain then stimulate the release of powerful neurochemicals into the blood which are then transported around the body. Molecules inhaled into the lungs may pass into the bloodstream and be disseminated in the same way.

When rubbed or massaged into the skin, essential oils will permeate the pores and hair follicles. From here, they can readily pass into the tiny blood vessels known as capillaries by virtue of their molecular structure, and then travel around the body.

Once absorbed, the action of the oil depends upon its chemical constituents. Most essential oils are high in alcohols and esters, although a few contain a high concentration of phenols, aldehydes and ketones. The latter are powerful chemicals and their use should be avoided by all save the skilled professional.

Beneficial essential oils

Essential oils that are particularly beneficial for headaches include the following.

CHAMOMILE, ROMAN (*Chamaemelum nobile*) There are several varieties, but Roman chamomile is the essential oil of choice for home use. It is used by therapists to treat many skin complaints and promotes the healing of burns, cuts, bites and inflammations. It is also effective in allergic conditions and can have a beneficial effect on menstrual problems when used regularly in the bath. It seems to be effective in reducing stress and anxiety and problems such as headache, migraine and insomnia. As an analgesic, it is used in the treatment of earache, toothache, neuralgia and abscesses, and is popular for treating childhood illnesses. CAUTION: Chamomile is generally nontoxic and nonirritant, but may cause dermatitis in very sensitive individuals.

GERANIUM (*Pelargonium graveolens*) Geranium is an excellent 'all-round' oil, with a wide range of uses, but particularly good for headaches, menopausal problems and premenstrual tension. Its diuretic quality makes it a wise choice for fluid retention, and cellulitis and mastitis often respond well to it. For skin conditions and emotional disorders, it is a popular choice in the bath and in massage oil. Serious skin conditions often respond to its antiseptic and antifungal qualities. CAUTION: Generally nontoxic and nonirritant, it may cause contact dermatitis in hypersensitive individuals.

LAVENDER (*Lavendula vera*) The highly perfumed lavender is a native species of the Mediterranean but has long been popular as a garden plant in Britain and many other countries. It has antiseptic, tonic and relaxing properties, and the essential oil used in aromatherapy is obtained by subjecting the flowers to a process of steam distillation. It is considered to be one of the safest preparations and is used in the treatment of a wide range of disorders. Lavender is an appetite stimulant, an antispasmodic and a tonic. It is particularly effective in the treatment of minor burns and scalds, wounds, sores and varicose ulcers, and is generally one of the most versatile and widely used oils for healing. It also has a strong antiseptic effect and is employed in many cosmetic preparations and as an insect repellent. It is also used in the treatment of muscular aches and pains, respiratory problems, influenza, digestive problems, and genito-urinary problems such as cystitis and dysmenorrhoea. Its soothing effect is recommended for headaches and premenstrual tension. Lavender is a very safe oil and can even be applied undiluted to the skin.

MARJORAM, SWEET (*Origanum marjorana*) Marjoram can be extremely effective in reducing the pain and swelling of muscular damage, bruises and sprains, and arthritis, and for the treatment of headaches. It has an extremely hypnotic effect, which is useful in inducing sleep and calming emotions, especially when used in the bath. It can also be effective in menstrual problems. Marjoram is also a popular treatment for colds and coughs, bronchitis and asthma, and has a carminative and antispasmodic action on colic, constipation and flatulence. CAUTION: It should be avoided by pregnant women as it has a strong emmenagogic effect.

PEPPERMINT (*Mentha piperita*) Peppermint is a native plant of Europe with a long history of medicinal use dating back to the ancient civilisations of Egypt, Greece and Rome. Oil of peppermint is obtained by subjecting the flowering parts of the plant to a process of steam distillation. The essential oil of peppermint has a calming effect on the digestive tract and is excellent for the relief of indigestion, colic-type pains, nausea, travel and morning sickness. It is also anextremely gentle inhalation for asthma. It is cooling and refreshing, and useful in the treatment of colds, respiratory symptoms and headaches. Peppermint is widely used in remedies for colds and indigestion, as a food flavouring,especially in confectionery, and in toothpaste. CAUTION: Possibly irritant to sensitive skin – use in moderation always.

ROSE (*Rosa centifola*) Rose has a supremely feminine and deeply sensual aroma, and is the traditional mainstay of the perfume industry. Rose oil has a wonderful antidepressant effect that may be harnessed in body and face massages, baths or vaporisers to treat anxiety, stress and depression. It also has a gentle balancing effect on gynaecological disorders and is said to have aphrodisiac properties.

ROSEMARY (*Rosemarinus officinalis*) Rosemary has a wide application and is effective in the treatment of numerous complaints. Possessing a powerful aroma, rosemary is favoured as a decongestant in inhalation and an invigorating muscle-strengthening massage oil. Skin and hair problems can respond well to rosemary, and gargling with it will freshen the breath. Above all, rosemary seems to possess remarkable memory and concentration-enhancing properties. Other therapeutic uses are in alleviating headaches, digestive disorders and stress. CAUTION: Rosemary should be avoided during pregnancy and should not be used by anyone suffering from epilepsy.

SAGE (*Salvia officinalis*) Sage is a native plant of the northern coastal regions of the Mediterranean and has a long history of medicinal and culinary use dating back to the ancient civilisations of Greece and Rome. The essential oil used in aromatherapy is obtained by subjecting the dried leaves to a process of steam distillation. Sage has an expectorant effect when used in inhalations, and its astringent and cooling properties make it a popular choice as a tonic, an appetite stimulant and as a fever reducer. If used in a gargle or mouthwash, its antiseptic effects are beneficial to sore throats and mouth problems. It is also used to improve poor circulation, colds and viral infections, bronchitic and catarrhal complaints, rheumatism, arthritic pains, joint sprains and strains, and headaches. Sage is widely used as a flavouring in foods and in some household preparations and toiletries. CAUTION: Sage should be avoided during pregnancy and should not be used by anyone suffering from epilepsy.

Aromatherapy treatments

Many of the essential oils can be safely used at home and the basic techniques of use can soon be mastered. However, some should only be used by a trained aromatherapist and others must be avoided in certain conditions such as pregnancy. In some circumstances, massage is not considered to be advisable. It is wise to seek medical advice in the event of doubt or if the ailment is more than a minor one. Some treatments are described below.

Massage

Massage is the most familiar method of treatment associated with aromatherapy. Essential oils are able to penetrate through the skin and are taken into the body, exerting healing and beneficial influences on internal tissues and organs. The oils used for massage are first diluted by being mixed with a base oil and should never be applied directly to the skin in their pure form in case of an adverse allergic reaction.

An aromatherapist will 'design' an individual whole body massage based on an accurate history taken from the patient and much experience in the use of essential oils. The oils will be chosen specifically to match the temperament of the patient and also to deal with any particular medical or emotional problems which may be troubling him (or her). Although there is no substitute for a long, soothing aromatherapy massage given by an expert, massage techniques are not difficult to learn and can be carried out satisfactorily at home.

Basic techniques of massage

The following constitutes only a very basic guide to massage and is no substitute for a comprehensive aromamassage course. However, massage can be used to great benefit at home using the following simple movements and suggestions.

EFFLEURAGE This is the most often used therapy movement, and constitutes a simple, gentle stroking movement. Note that deep pressure should never be used by an untrained person. The strokes may be long or short, gentle or firm, but the whole hand should be used, always pushing the blood towards the heart, thus promoting venous return. This stroke promotes muscle relaxation and soothes the nerve endings.

PETRISSAGE In petrissage, the flesh is gently rolled between the thumbs and fingers in a movement not unlike kneading dough. This technique is best used on the back and on fatty areas. The idea is to stimulate the circulation and lymphatic flow and thereby increase the rate of toxin expulsion.

HEAD MASSAGE Put a little of the essential massage oil on the fingertips and massage in circular movements over the scalp and temples.

MASSAGE FOR TENSION HEADACHES AND MIGRAINE Working from the base of the neck and scalp for a few moments, use effleurage strokes firmly, again with the chosen oil(s) on the fingertips.

NECK MASSAGE Neck massage should be carried out with the patient sitting on a chair with some support in front. Working around the base of the neck and scalp, use small upward and outward circular movements. Move slowly up, down and around the sides of the neck, alternating firm and gentle movements.

SHOULDER MASSAGE Using gentle anticlockwise effleurage movements, stroke firmly from the shoulders to the neck.

Inhalation

Inhalation is thought to be the most direct and rapid means of treatment. This is because the molecules of the volatile essential oil act directly on the olfactory organs and are immediately perceived by the brain. A popular method is the time-honoured one of steam inhalation, in which a few drops of essential oil are added to hot water in a bowl. The person sits with his (or her) face above the mixture and covers the head, face and bowl with a towel so that the vapours do not escape. This can be repeated up to three times a day but should not be undertaken by people suffering from asthma. Some essential oils can be applied directly to a handkerchief or onto a pillow and the vapours inhaled in this way.

Steam inhalation with essential oils constitutes a wonderful, time-honoured way of alleviating the symptoms of colds and flu, and can also be beneficial to greasy skins. Steam inhalations should, however, be avoided by asthmatics unless under direction from a medical practitioner, as the steam can occasionally irritate the lungs.

Bathing and showering

Most people have experienced the benefits of relaxing in a hot bath to which a proprietary perfumed preparation has been added. Most of these preparations contain the same essential oils that are used in aromatherapy. The addition of a number of drops of an essential oil to the bath water is soothing and relaxing, easing aches and pains, and can also have a stimulating effect, banishing tiredness and restoring energy. In addition, there is the added benefit of inhaling the vapours of the oil as they evaporate from the hot water. Add 5 to 10 drops of essential oil to the bath water after the water has been drawn, then close the door to retain the aromatic vapours. The choice of oils is entirely up to the individual, depending on the desired effect, although those with sensitive skins are advised to have the oils already diluted in a base oil prior to bathing.

Bathing in essential oils can stimulate and revive or relax and sedate depending on the oils selected: rosemary and pine can have a soothing effect on tired or aching limbs, chamomile and lavender are popular for relieving insomnia and anxiety, etc. A similar effect (although obviously not quite as relaxing) can be achieved whilst showering by soaking a wet sponge in an essential oil mix, then rubbing it over the body under the warm spray.

Compresses

Compresses are effective in the treatment of a variety of muscular and rheumatic aches and pains as well as bruises and headaches. To prepare a compress, add 5 drops of oil to a small bowl of water. Cold water should be used wherever fever or acute pain or hot swelling require treatment, whereas the water should be hot if the pain is chronic. Soak a piece of absorbent material in the solution. Squeeze out excess moisture (although the compress should remain fairly wet) and secure in position with a bandage or cling film. For acute pain, the compress should be renewed when it has reached blood temperature, otherwise it should be left in position for a minimum of 2 hours and preferably overnight. If fever is present, the compress should be changed frequently.

Around the home

There are a variety of ways in which your home can be enhanced by the use of essential oils. Fragrancers, pomanders, ring burners and diffusers can all be used in conjunction with essential oils to impart a wonderful scent to a room. (Essential oils should be put into water and vaporised and *not* burned as they are inflammable. Follow the instructions on ring burners carefully and never put essential oils directly onto a hot light bulb.) Most essential oils also have antimicrobial properties which make them extremely useful when the occupants of the room are suffering from colds and flu. Oils such as myrtle and eucalyptus also seem to have a soothing effect on coughs and can be used in the bedroom where they will release their aroma throughout the night.

Fragrancers, pomanders, and ring burners can all be purchased quite cheaply from shops and indeed make very welcome gifts, but it is not necessary to use any extra equipment to benefit from essential oils in the home. By adding a few drops of essential oil to a bowl of water, or by soaking a cotton ball in the oil and placing it in a warm place, the same effect can be achieved. You can also sprinkle logs and twigs before placing them on the fire or barbecue to create a soothing aroma.

In case of colds or flu, a bowl of water is actually preferable as it has a humidifying effect on the air. Also, 3 or 4 drops of an appropriate essential oil, such as eucalyptus or cypress, sprinkled on a handkerchief can be inhaled periodically to alleviate the worst symptoms of sinusitis, colds and headaches. Similarly, 2 to 3 drops of a relaxing essential oil on the pillow at night can help to alleviate insomnia.

Conditions that may benefit from aromatherapy

A wide range of conditions and disorders may benefit from aromatherapy which is considered to be a gentle treatment suitable for all age groups. It is especially beneficial for long-term chronic conditions, and the use of essential oils is believed by therapists to prevent the development of some illnesses. Aromatherapy may relieve tension headaches, painful limbs, muscles and joints due to arthritic or rheumatic disorders, respiratory complaints, digestive disorders, skin conditions, throat and mouth infections, urinary tract infections and problems affecting the hair and scalp. Also, period pains, burns, insect bites and stings, high blood pressure, feverishness, menopausal symptoms, poor circulation and gout can benefit from aromatherapy. Aromatherapy is of great benefit in relieving stress and stress-related symptoms such as anxiety, insomnia and depression.

Consulting a professional aromatherapist

Aromatherapy is a holistic approach to healing hence the practitioner endeavours to build up a complete picture of the patient and his (or her) lifestyle, nature and family circumstances, as well as noting the symptoms which need to be treated.

Depending upon the picture obtained, the aromatherapist decides upon the essential oil or oils that are most suitable and likely to prove most helpful in the circumstances that prevail. Aromatherapists are able to draw on their wide-ranging knowledge and experience and many offer a massage and/or instruction on the use of the selected oils at home.

Chapter 18

BIOFEEDBACK

Biofeedback essentially involves training individuals to recognise, and hence try to alter and control, various bodily rhythms that are indicative of internal stress or disorder. Various types of monitoring equipment, some of it highly technical and linked to computers, may be employed to help the signals from the body to be detected and translated into a form that can be understood. For example, stress reactions that result from the release of the hormone, adrenaline, include a raised heartbeat, increased electrical conductance in the skin, a slowing down of digestive processes and sweating. These changes can be monitored with various types of devices and an individual can learn to control and minimise his (or her) stress reaction by employing relaxation techniques. If the person is linked to the machine, the successful effects of relaxation are made apparent and, in time, the individual can be trained to recognise stress and to use the technique to counter it without the need of any equipment.

Biofeedback is helpful for people suffering from various chronic, painful conditions as well as psychological and anxiety disorders. As has been seen, headaches and migraines are associated with high levels of stress, anxiety and muscular tension, and for some individuals several biofeedback techniques can be helpful, including the relaxation method described above and, also, a technique called electro-myographic feedback or EMG. This method provides a visible measure of muscular tension, for example in the neck, and gives the sufferer training in how to recognise tightened muscles and, more importantly, the relaxation techniques that will help to alleviate the tension.

Chapter 19

CHIROPRACTIC

Origins

The word 'chiropractic' originates from two Greek words: *kheir*, which means 'hand', and *praktikos*, which means 'practical'. A school of chiropractic was established in about 1895 by a healer called Daniel Palmer (1845–1913). He was able to cure a man's deafness that had occurred when he bent down and felt a bone click. Upon examination Palmer discovered that some bones of the man's spine had become displaced. After successful manipulation the man regained his hearing. Palmer formed the opinion that if there was any displacement in the skeleton this could affect the function of nerves, either increasing or decreasing their action and thereby resulting in a malfunction, i.e. a disease.

Conditions that may benefit from chiropractic

Chiropractic is used to relieve pain by manipulation and to correct any problems that are present in joints and muscles but especially the spine. Like osteopathy, no use is made of surgery or drugs. If there are any spinal disorders, they can cause widespread problems elsewhere in the body, such as the hip, leg or arm, and can also initiate lumbago, sciatica, a slipped disc or other back problems. It is even possible that spinal problems can result in seemingly unrelated problems such as catarrh, migraine, asthma, constipation, stress, etc.

However, the majority of a chiropractor's patients suffer mainly from neck and back pain and headaches. People suffering from neck pain and headaches as a result of whiplash injuries sustained in car accidents commonly seek the help of a chiropractor. The whiplash effect is caused when the head is violently wrenched either forwards or backwards at the time of impact. Where headaches are concerned, it is often the case that tension is the underlying cause as it makes the neck muscles contract. Athletes can also obtain relief from injuries such as tennis elbow, pulled muscles, injured ligaments and sprains, etc. As well as the normal methods of manipulating joints, the chiropractor may decide it is necessary to use applications of ice or heat to relieve the injury, as well as massage.

Children can also benefit from treatment by a chiropractor, as there may be some slight accident that occurs in their early years that can reappear in adult life in the form of back pain. It can easily happen, for example, when a child learns to walk and bumps into furniture, or when a baby falls out of a cot. This could result in some damage to the spine that will show only in adult life when a person experiences back pain. At birth, a baby's neck may be injured or the spine may be strained if the use of forceps is necessary, and this can result in headaches and neck problems as he (or she) grows to maturity. This early type of injury could also account for what is known as 'growing pains', when the real problem is actually damage that has been done to the bones or muscles. If a parent has any worries it is best to consult a doctor and it is possible that the child will be recommended to see a qualified chiropractor. To avoid any problems in adult life, chiropractors recommend that children have occasional examinations to detect any damage or displacement in bones and muscles.

As well as babies and children, adults of all ages can benefit from chiropractic. There are some people who regularly take painkillers for painful joints or back pain, but this does not deal with the root cause of the pain, only the symptoms that are produced. Many pregnant women experience backache at some stage during their pregnancy because of the extra weight that is placed on the spine, and they also may find it difficult keeping their balance. At the time of giving birth, changes take place in the pelvis and joints at the bottom of the spine and this can be a cause of back pain. Lifting and carrying babies, if not done correctly, can also damage the spine and thereby make the back painful.

Treatment

It is essential that any chiropractor is fully qualified and registered with the relevant professional association. At the initial visit, a patient will be asked for details of his (or her) case history, including the present problem, and during the examination painful and tender areas will be noted and joints will be checked to see whether they are functioning correctly or not. X-rays are frequently used by chiropractors since they can show signs of bone disease, fractures or arthritis as well as the spine's condition. After the initial visit, any treatment will normally begin as soon as the patient has been informed of the chiropractor's diagnosis. If it has been decided that chiropractic therapy will not be of any benefit, the patient will be advised accordingly.

For treatment, underwear and/or a robe will be worn, and the patient will either lie, sit or stand on a specially designed couch. Chiropractors use their hands in a skilful way to effect the different manipulative techniques. For example, if it is decided that manipulation is necessary to treat a painful lumbar joint, the patient will need to lie on his (or her) side. The upper and lower spine will then be rotated manually but in opposite ways. This manipulation will have the effect of partially locking the joint that is being treated, and the upper leg is usually flexed to aid the procedure. The vertebra that is immediately below or above the joint will then be felt by the chiropractor, and the combination of how the patient is lying, coupled with gentle pressure applied by the chiropractor's hand, will move the joint to its furthest extent of normal movement. There will then be a very quick push applied on the vertebra, which results in its movement being extended further than normal, ensuring that full use of the joint is regained. This is due to the muscles that surround the joint being suddenly stretched, which has the effect of relaxing the muscles of the spine that work upon the joint. This alteration should cause the joint to be able to be used more naturally and should not be a painful procedure.

There can be a variety of effects felt after treatment – some patients may feel sore or stiff, or may ache some time after the treatment, while others will experience the lifting of pain at once. In some cases there may be a need for multiple treatments, perhaps four or more, before improvement is felt. On the whole, problems that have been troubling a patient for a considerable time (chronic) will need more therapy than anything that occurs quickly and is very painful (acute).

There is quite a small number of chiropractors in the UK (although their numbers are increasing) but there is a degree of contact and liaison between them and doctors. It is generally accepted that chiropractic is an effective remedy for bone and muscular problems, and the majority of doctors would be happy to accept a chiropractor's diagnosis and treatment, although the treatment of any general diseases, such as diabetes or asthma, would not be viewed in the same manner.

Chapter 20

CRANIAL OSTEOPATHY

Cranial osteopathy is a refined, gentle and specialised branch of osteopathy (*see* **Osteopathy** on page 208) concentrated upon the head although it aims to relieve stresses and strains that may be present in any part of the body. A cranial osteopath is able to use his (or her) fingers to feel a subtle movement called the cranial rhythm or involuntary motion and this is present in the cerebrospinal fluid in the brain and spinal cord. Disorders and stresses anywhere in the body can disrupt the cranial rhythm causing blockages that may be very small in amplitude and it is this that the cranial osteopath is able to detect. Practitioners compare the patient's cranial rhythm to one that is considered ideal. The cranial rhythm was first described by William G. Sutherland in the 1920s and further research during the 1960s and 70s has yielded more information on the manner in which it operates.

Cranial osteopathy involves applying very gentle pressure to the sutures of the skull and it can be used on people of all ages, from young infants to the elderly. The aim is to remove any blockage or irregularity in the flow of the cranial rhythm, thereby alleviating the disorder for which the person has sought treatment. Headaches, migraines, musculo-skeletal pains, especially in the face, neck and spine, hearing problems, sinusitis, chronic ear infections, problems associated with cerebral palsy, and learning and behavioural disorders in children are all conditions which may benefit from this form of therapy.

Chapter 21

HERBALISM

The nature of herbalism

Herbalism is sometimes maligned as a collection of home-made remedies to be applied in a placebo fashion to one symptom or another, provided the ailment is not too serious and provided there is a powerful chemical wonder-drug at the ready to suppress any 'real' symptoms. We often forget, however, that botanical medicine provides a complete system of healing and disease prevention. It is the oldest and most natural form of medicine. Its record of efficacy and safety spans centuries and covers every country worldwide. Because herbal medicine is holistic medicine, it is, in fact, able to look beyond the symptoms to the underlying systemic imbalance; when skilfully applied by a trained practitioner, herbal medicine offers very real and permanent solutions to concrete problems, many of them seemingly intractable to pharmaceutical intervention.

The origins and history of herbalism

Early civilisations

The medicinal use of herbs is said to be as old as mankind itself. In early civilisations, food and medicine were linked and many plants were eaten for their health-giving properties. In ancient Egypt, the slave workers were given a daily ration of garlic to help fight off the many fevers and infections that were common at that time. The first written records of herbs and their beneficial properties were compiled by the ancient Egyptians – most of our knowledge and use of herbs can be traced back to the Egyptian priests who practised herbal medicine. Records dating back to 1500 BC listed medicinal herbs, including caraway and cinnamon.

The ancient Greeks and Romans also carried out herbal medicine, and as they invaded new lands their doctors encountered new herbs and introduced herbs such as rosemary or lavender into new areas. China and India also have a history of herbal medicine. In Britain, the use of herbs developed along with the establishment of monasteries around the country, each of which had its own herb garden for use in treating both the monks and the local people. In some areas, particularly Wales and Scotland, Druids and other Celtic healers are thought to have had an oral tradition of herbalism, where medicine was mixed with religion and ritual.

The first publications

Over time, these healers and their knowledge led to the writing of the first 'herbals', which rapidly rose in importance and distribution upon the advent of the printing press in the fifteenth century. John Parkinson of London wrote a herbal around 1630, listing useful plants.

Many herbalists set up their own apothecary shops, including the famous Nicholas Culpepper (1616–1654) whose most famous work is *The Complete Herbal and English Physician, Enlarged*, published in 1649. Then in 1812, Henry Potter started a business supplying herbs and dealing in leeches. By this time a huge amount of traditional knowledge and folklore on medicinal herbs was available from Britain, Europe, the Middle East,

Asia and the Americas. This prompted Potter to write *Potter's Encyclopaedia of Botanical Drugs and Preparations*, which is still published today.

The decline of herbal medicine

It was in this period that scientifically inspired conventional medicine rose in popularity, sending herbal medicine into a decline. But in rural areas herbal medicine continued to thrive in local folklore, traditions and practices. In 1864 the National Association (later Institute) of Medical Herbalists was established, to organise training of herbal medicine practitioners and to maintain standards of practice. From 1864 until the early part of the twentieth century, the Institute fought attempts to ban herbal medicine and over time public interest in herbal medicine has increased, particularly over the last 20 years.

This move away from synthetic drugs is partly due to possible side effects, bad publicity, and, in some instances, a mistrust of the medical and pharmacological industries. The more natural appearance of herbal remedies has led to its growing support and popularity. Herbs from America have been incorporated into common remedies, and scientific research into herbs and their active ingredients has confirmed their healing power and enlarged the range of medicinal herbs used today.

The relevance of herbal medicine today

Herbal medicine can be viewed as the precursor of modern pharmacology, but today it continues as an effective and more natural method of treating and preventing illness. Globally, herbal medicine is 3 to 4 times more commonly practised than conventional medicine.

Nowhere is the efficacy of herbalism more evident than in problems related to the nervous system. Stress, anxiety, tension and depression are intimately connected with most illness. Few health practitioners would argue over the influence of nervous anxiety in pathology. Nervous tension is generally acknowledged by doctors to contribute to duodenal and gastric ulceration, ulcerative colitis, irritable bowel syndrome and many other gut-related pathologies.

We know also, from physiology, that when a person is depressed, the secretion of hydrochloric acid – one of the main digestive juices – is also reduced so that digestion and absorption are rendered less efficient. Anxiety, on the other hand, can lead to the release of adrenaline and stimulate the overproduction of hydrochloric acid and result in a state of acidity that may exacerbate the pain of an inflamed ulcer. In fact, whenever the voluntary nervous system (our conscious anxiety) interferes with the autonomic processes (the automatic nervous regulation that in health is never made conscious), illness is the result.

Herbalists rely on their knowledge of botanical remedies to rectify this type of human malfunction. The medical herbalist will treat a stubborn dermatological problem using 'alternatives' specific to the skin problem, and then apply circulatory stimulants to aid in the removal of toxins from the area, with remedies to reinforce other organs of elimination, such as the liver and kidneys. Under such natural treatment, free of any discomforting side effects, the patient can feel confident and relaxed – perhaps for the first time in many months.

Curiously, this is an approach that has never been taken up by orthodox medicine. There, the usual treatment of skin problems involves suppression of symptoms with steroids. However, the use of conventional antihistamines or benzodiazepines often achieves less lasting benefit to the patient because of the additional burden of side effects, such as drowsiness, increased toxicity, and long-term drug dependence.Herbs, on the other hand, because they are organic substances and not manmade synthetic molecules, possess an affinity for the human organism. They are extremely efficient in balancing the nervous system.

Restoring a sense of wellbeing and relaxation is necessary for optimum health and for the process of self-healing. Naturally, the choice of a treatment should be based upon a thorough health assessment and the experience and training of a qualified herbal practitioner. The herbalist will then prepare and prescribe herbal remedies in a variety of different forms, such as infusions, loose teas, suppositories, inhalants, lotions, tinctures, tablets and pills. Many of these preparations are available for home use from chemists, health shops and mail-order suppliers.

Forms of herbal preparations

CAPSULE A capsule is a gelatine container for swallowing and holding oils or balsams that would otherwise be difficult to administer due to their unpleasant taste or smell. For example, it is used for cod liver oil and castor oil.

DECOCTION A decoction is prepared using cut, bruised or ground bark and roots placed into a stainless steel or enamel pan (not aluminium) with cold water poured on. The mixture is boiled for 20 to 30 minutes, cooled and strained. It is best drunk when warm.

HERBAL DRESSING A herbal dressing may be a compress or poultice. A compress is made of cloth or cotton wool soaked in cold or warm herbal decoctions or infusions while a poultice can be made with fresh or dried herbs. Bruised fresh herbs are applied directly to the affected area and dried herbs are made into a paste with water and placed on gauze on the required area. Both dressings are very effective in easing pain, swelling and inflammation of the skin and tissues.

INFUSION An infusion is a liquid made from ground or bruised roots, bark, herbs or seeds, by pouring boiling water onto the herb and leaving it to stand for 10 to 30 minutes, possibly stirring the mixture occasionally. The resultant liquid is strained and used. Cold infusions may be made if the active principles are yielded from the herb without heat. Today, infusions may be packaged into tea-bags for convenience.

LIQUID EXTRACT A liquid extract, if correctly made, is the most concentrated fluid form in which herbal drugs may be obtained and, as such, is very popular and convenient. Each herb is treated by various means dependent upon the individual properties of the herb, e.g. cold percolation, high pressure, and evaporation by heat in a vacuum. These extracts are commonly held in a household stock of domestic remedies.

PESSARY A pessary is similar to a suppository, but it is used in female complaints to apply a preparation to the walls of the vagina and cervix.

PILL The pill is probably the best known and most widely used herbal preparation. It is normally composed of concentrated extracts and alkaloids, in combination with active crude drugs. The pill may be coated with sugar or another pleasant-tasting substance that is readily soluble in the stomach.

SOLID EXTRACT A solid extract is prepared by evaporating the fresh juices or strong infusions of herbal drugs to the consistency of honey. It may also be prepared from an alcoholic tincture base. It is used mainly to produce pills, plasters, ointments and compressed tablets.

SUPPOSITORY A suppository is a small cone of a convenient and easily soluble base with herbal extracts added, which is used to apply medicines to the rectum. It is very effective in the treatment of piles.

TABLET A tablet is made by compressing drugs into a small compass. It is more easily administered and has a quicker action as it dissolves more rapidly in the stomach.

TINCTURE A tincture is the most prescribed form of herbal medicine. It is based on alcohol and, as such, removes certain active principles from herbs that will not dissolve in water, or in the presence of heat. The tincture produced is long-lasting, highly concentrated and only needs to be taken in small doses for beneficial effects. The ground or chopped dried herb is placed in a container with 40% alcohol, such as gin or vodka, and left for 2 weeks. The tincture is then decanted into a dark bottle and sealed before use.

Herbal preparations for headaches

Herbal preparations that are particularly useful for treating stress and headaches include the following:

ANEMONE, WOOD (*Anemone nemorosa*)
Common name: crowfoot, windflower, smell fox.
Occurrence: found in woods and thickets across the UK.
Parts used: the root, leaves and juice.
Medicinal uses: this species of plant is much less widely used than it has been previously. It used to be good for headaches, lethargy, and eye inflammation.
Administered as: decoction, fresh leaves and root, ointment.

BALM (*Melissa officinalis*)
Common name: sweet balm, lemon balm, honey plant, cure-all.
Occurrence: a common garden plant across the UK, which was naturalised into southern England at a very early period.
Parts used: the herb.
Medicinal uses: as a carminative, diaphoretic, or febrifuge. It can be made into a cooling tea for fever patients and balm is often used in combination with other herbs to treat colds and fever.
Administered as: an infusion.

CAYENNE (*Capsicum minimum, Capsicum frutescens*)
Common name: African pepper, chillies, bird pepper.
Occurrence: native to Zanzibar but is now cultivated in most tropical and subtropical countries, e.g. Sierra Leone, Japan and Madagascar.
Parts used: the fruit, both fresh and dried.
Medicinal uses: stimulant, tonic, carminative, rubefacient. It is possibly the purest and best stimulant in herbal medicine. It produces natural warmth and helps the blood circulation, and eases weakness of the stomach and intestines. Cayenne is added to tonics and is said to ward off disease and can prevent development of colds and fevers.
Administered as: powdered fruit, tincture, capsules, dietary item.

CHAMOMILE (*Anthemis nobilis*)
Common name: Roman chamomile, double chamomile, manzanilla (Spanish), maythen (Saxon).
Occurrence: a low growing plant found wild across the UK.
Parts used: the flowers and herb. The active principles are a volatile oil, anthemic acid, tannic acid and a glucoside.
Medicinal uses: tonic, stomachic, anodyne and antispas-

modic. An infusion of chamomile tea is an extremely effective remedy for hysterical and nervous afflictions in women, as well as an emmenagogue. Chamomile has a powerful soothing and sedative effect which is harmless. A tincture is used to cure diarrhoea in children and it is used with purgatives to prevent griping, and as a tonic it helps dropsy. Externally, it can be applied alone or with other herbs as a poultice to relieve pain, swellings, inflammation and neuralgia. Its strong antiseptic properties make it invaluable for reducing swelling of the face due to abscess or injury. As a lotion, the flowers are good for resolving toothache and earache. The herb itself is an ingredient in herb beers. The use of chamomile can be dated back to ancient Egyptian times when they dedicated the plant to the sun because of its extensive healing properties.

Administered as: decoction, infusion, fluid extract and essential oil.

FEVERFEW (*Chrysanthemum parthenium*)
Common name: featherfew, featherfoil, flirtwort, bachelor's buttons, pyrethrum parthenium.
Occurrence: a wild hedgerow plant found in many areas of Europe and the UK.
Parts used: the herb.
Medicinal uses: as an aperient, carminative, bitter, stimulant, and emmenagogue. It is employed in hysterical complaints, nervousness and low spirits as a general tonic. A decoction is useful in easing coughs, wheezing and difficult breathing. Earache was relieved by a cold infusion while a tincture of feverfew eased the pain and swelling caused after insect or vermin bites. The herb was planted around dwellings to purify the atmosphere and ward off disease. Today, it is used to prevent or ease migraines or headaches.

Administered as: warm or cold infusion, poultice, tincture, decoction.

MARJORAM (*Origanum vulgare*)
Common names: sweet marjoram, knotted marjoram and pot marjoram.
Occurrence: generally distributed over Asia, Europe and North Africa and also found freely in the UK.
Parts used: the herb and volatile oil.
Medicinal uses: the oil has stimulant, carminative, diaphoretic, mildly tonic and emmenagogue qualities. As a warm infusion, it is used to produce perspiration and bring out the spots of measles as well as giving relief from spasms, colic and dyspeptic pain. The oil has been used externally as a rubefacient and liniment, and on cotton wool placed next to an aching tooth it relieves the pain. The dried herb may be utilised as a hot poultice for swellings, rheumatism and colic, while an infusion of the fresh plant will ease a nervous headache.
Administered as: essential oil, poultice and infusion.

ROSEMARY (*Rosmarinus officinalis*)
Common name: polar plant, compass-weed, compass plant, romero, *Rosmarinus coronarium*.
Occurrence: native to the dry hills of the Mediterranean, from Spain westward to Turkey. A common garden plant in the UK, cultivated prior to the Norman Conquest.
Parts used: the herb and root. Oil of rosemary is distilled from the plant tops and used medicinally. Rosemary contains tannic acid, a bitter principle, resin and a volatile oil.
Medicinal uses: tonic, astringent, diaphoretic, stimulant. The essential oil is also stomachic, nervine and carminative and cures many types of headache. It is mainly applied externally as a hair lotion which is said to prevent baldness

and the formation of dandruff. The oil is used externally as a rubefacient and is added to liniments for fragrance and stimulant properties. Rosemary tea can remove headache, colic, colds and nervous diseases and may also lift nervous depression.

Administered as: infusion, essential oil and lotion.

RUE (*Ruta graveolens*)

Common name: herb of grace, garden rue, herbygrass, ave-grace.

Occurrence: indigenous to southern Europe and was introduced into the UK by the Romans.

Parts used: the herb. The herb is covered by glands which contain a volatile oil. The oil is composed of methylnonylketone, limonene, cineole, a crystalline substance called rutin and several acids. The plant also contains several alkaloids including fagarine and arborinine as well as coumarins.

Medicinal uses: stimulant, antispasmodic, emmenagogue, irritant, rubefacient. This is a very powerful herb and the dose administered should be kept low. It is useful in treating coughs, croup, colic, flatulence, hysteria and it is particularly good against strained eyes and headaches caused by eyestrain. An infusion of the herb is good for nervous indigestion, heart palpitations, nervous headaches and to expel worms. The chemical, rutin, strengthens weak blood vessels and aids varicose veins. In Chinese medicine, rue is a specific for insect and snake bites. When made into an ointment, rue is effective in gouty and rheumatic pains, sprained and bruised tendons and chilblains. The bruised leaves irritate and blister the skin and so can ease sciatica. This herb should not be used in pregnancy as the volatile oil, alkaloids and coumarins in the plant all stimulate the uterus and strongly promote menstrual bleeding. When a fresh leaf is chewed, it flavours the mouth and relieves headache, giddiness or any hysterical spasms quickly.

Administered as: fresh leaf, volatile oil, ointment, infusion, decoction, tea, expressed

VALERIAN (*Valeriana officinalis*)

Common name: all-heal, great wild valerian, amantilla, setwall, sete-wale, capon's tail.

Occurrence: found throughout Europe and northern Asia. It is common in England in marshy thickets, riverbanks and ditches.

Parts used: the root, which contains a volatile oil, two alkaloids called chatarine and valerianine as well as several unidentified compounds.

Medicinal uses: a powerful nervine, stimulant, carminative anodyne and antispasmodic herb. The expressed juice of the fresh root has been used as a narcotic in insomnia and as an anticonvulsant in epilepsy. The oil of valerian is of use against cholera and in strengthening the eyesight. A herbal compound containing valerian was given to civilians during the Second World War, to reduce the effects of stress caused by repeated air raids and to minimise damage to health.

Administered as: fluid and solid extract, tincture, oil, expressed juice.

Soothing herbal drinks

Warm milk and honey

A drink of warm milk and honey is an ideal drink to take at bedtime, perhaps with a dash of cinnamon. It will help you relax and ward off insomnia.

Hop tea

Three hop cones, or heads, infused in a cup of boiling water whenever you begin to feel excessively tense, is a marvellous remedy for anxiety and insomnia.

A soothing herb tea to sustain a feeling of equilibrium

    25g (1 oz) each dried chamomile flowers, lime flowers,
        hibiscus blossoms and marigold flowers
    15g (½ oz) each dried peppermint leaves and vervain
    1 teaspoon whole fenugreek seeds
    100g (4 oz) Lapsang Souchong tea

Mix all the ingredients together and store in a dark airtight container.

Use 1 teaspoon of the tea mixture to 300 ml (½ pint) of boiling water in a teapot and leave to infuse for 5 minutes before straining and serving with a slice of lemon and a teaspoon of honey if desired.

This is a very calming tea that soothes feelings of anxiety. It also helps to clear your head and settle an upset tummy. One cup taken morning and night will promote a feeling of wellbeing.

Another calming tea, especially good for the nerves

    1 teaspoon each grated valerian root and dried mint
    ½ teaspoon each dried chamomile and lavender flowers
    600 ml (1 pint) boiling water

Infuse the dry ingredients in the water for 15 minutes then strain and take a glass 3 times a day for 1 week only.

Two tonic teas to sip when feeling depressed

Sip either:

2 teaspoons of dandelion and 1 teaspoon of basil infused in 600 ml (1 pint) of boiling water

or

2 teaspoons each of nettle, basil and melissa infused in 600 ml (1 pint) of boiling water.

A tonic tea to relieve stress and anxiety

1 tablespoon each fresh dandelion and nettle tops
1 teaspoon each fresh blackcurrant and borage leaves
600 ml (1 pint) boiling water

Steep the greenery in the water for 5 minutes. Strain and drink with lemon and honey.

Chapter 22

HOMEOPATHY

The homeopathic approach

The aim of homeopathy is to cure an illness or disorder by treating the whole person rather than merely concentrating on a set of symptoms. Hence, in homeopathy the approach is holistic, and the overall state of health of the patient, especially his (or her) emotional and psychological wellbeing, is regarded as being significant. A homeopath notes the symptoms that the person wishes to have cured but also takes time to discover other signs or indications of disorder that the patient may regard as being less important. The reasoning behind this is that illness is a sign of disorder or imbalance within the body. It is believed that the whole 'make-up' of a person determines, to a great extent, the type of disorders to which that individual is prone and the symptoms likely to occur. A homeopathic remedy must be suitable both for the symptoms and the characteristics and temperament of the patient. Hence, two patients with the same illness may be offered different remedies according to their individual natures. One remedy may also be used to treat different groups of symptoms or ailments.

Like cures like

Homeopathic remedies are based on the concept that 'like cures like', an ancient philosophy that can be traced back to the fifth century BC, when it was formulated by Hippocrates. In the early 1800s, this idea awakened the interest of a German doctor, Samuel Hahnemann, who believed that the medical practices at the time were too harsh and tended to hinder rather than aid healing. Hahnemann observed that a treatment for malaria, based on an extract of cinchona bark (quinine), actually produced symptoms of this disease when taken in a small dose by a healthy person. Further extensive studies convinced him that the production of symptoms was the body's way of combating illness. Hence, to give a minute dose of a substance that stimulated the symptoms of an illness in a healthy person could be used to fight that illness in someone who was sick. Hahnemann conducted numerous trials (called 'provings'), giving minute doses of substances to healthy people and recording the symptoms produced. Eventually, these very dilute remedies were given to people with illnesses, often with encouraging results.

Homeopathic remedies

Modern homeopathy is based on the work of Hahnemann, and the medicines derived from plant, mineral and animal sources are used in extremely dilute amounts. Indeed, it is believed that the curative properties are enhanced by each dilution because impurities that might cause unwanted side effects are lost. Substances used in homeopathy are first soaked in alcohol to extract their essential ingredients. This initial solution, called the 'mother tincture', is diluted successively either by factors of ten (called the 'decimal scale' and designated X) or 100 (the 'centesimal scale' and designated C). Each dilution is shaken vigorously before further ones are made, and this is thought to make the properties more powerful by adding energy at each stage while impurities are removed. The thorough shakings of each dilution are said to energise, or 'potentiate', the medicine. The remedies are made into tablets or may be used in the form of ointment, solutions, powders, suppositories, etc. High potency (i.e. more dilute) remedies are used for severe symptoms and lower potency (less dilute) for milder ones.

The homeopathic view is that during the process of healing, symptoms are redirected from more important to less important body systems. It is also held that healing is from innermost to outermost parts of the body and that more recent symptoms disappear first, this being known as the 'law of direction of cure'. Occasionally, symptoms may worsen initially when a homeopathic remedy is taken, but this is usually short-lived and is known as a 'healing crisis'. It is taken to indicate a change and that improvement is likely to follow. Usually, with a homeopathic remedy, an improvement is noticed fairly quickly although this depends upon the nature of the ailment, the health, age and wellbeing of the patient, and the potency of the remedy.

Potency table for homeopathic medicines

The centesimal scale

1C = 1/100	(1/100^1) of mother tincture
2C = 1/10 000	(1/100^2) of mother tincture
3C = ¹⁄₁ 000 000	(1/100^3) of mother tincture
6C = ¹⁄₁ 000 000 000 000	(1/100^6) of mother tincture

The decimal scale

1X = 1/10	(1/10^1) of mother tincture
2X = 1/100	(1/10^2) of mother tincture
6X = ¹⁄₁ 000 000	(1/10^6) of mother tincture

Treatment

A first homeopathic consultation is likely to last about an hour so that the specialist can obtain a full picture of the patient's medical history and personal circumstances. On the basis of this information, the homeopathic doctor decides on an appropriate remedy and potency (which is usually 6C). Subsequent consultations are generally shorter, and full advice is given on how to store and take the medicine. It is widely accepted that homeopathic remedies are safe and nonaddictive, but they are covered by the legal requirements governing all medicines and should be obtained from a recognised source.

Homeopathic medicines for headaches

Homeopathic medicines are available over-the-counter but it is preferable for you to receive guidance from a homeopathic practitioner. Dosage and frequency of the preparations will vary and you may be using only one medicine or a combination. The following homeopathic medicines may be suggested as possible remedies for headaches and migraine:

BELLADONNA is for throbbing, pounding headaches where the sufferer is sensitive to noise and lights.

NUX VOMICA is a common headache remedy often indicated for headaches related to food triggers or alcohol.

SILICEA for migraines triggered by hormones or those related to exertion.

IGNATIA for headaches related to grief or depression.

ARNICA is recommended for headaches related to head trauma or injury.

IRIS for intense migraines, particularly those with aura and other visual disturbances.

SPIGELIA for sharp, painful throbbing headaches.

LACHESIS for excruciating migraines, with pain often on the left side.

SANGUINARIA is used for migraines that are felt mostly on the right side of the head, with painful sensitivity to lights and sounds.

Chapter 23

MEDITATION AND YOGA

Meditation

Meditation is the art of transcending everyday thought processes – if only for a very short period of time, our minds briefly escape the tyranny of worry, and we begin to get a sense of who we truly are and what we truly feel. Meditation also has physical benefits. By enabling us to access inner calm, it helps us to release tension and to alleviate the stress that is being linked to more and more physical ailments, from headaches and migraine to high blood pressure. Also, experts in pain management believe that a combination of both medical and behavioural medicine is the most effective way of managing pain, including headaches. Behavioural medicine trains us to become aware of the power of our minds and emotions on our health and to use this power to alleviate pain and improve our quality of life.

In its simplest form, meditation is nothing more than allowing the mind to be lulled by a simple repetitive sensation – waves lapping on the beach, the tinkling of water from a fountain, repeating a word or sound over and over again, even something as mundane as the sound of machinery. Any of these, and countless others, can be used as something on which the mind focuses itself completely, thus putting worry and anxiety on the back burner for a while and alleviating pain. We have all done this naturally at some time or another: you may have gazed into a beautiful sunset and become absorbed in the flames of colour, or been seduced by the lapping of waves on the seashore and the heat from the sun. Children are much better at this than adults. Think of a child, bent over a half-finished painting, and think of the number of times he (or she) has to be called before they hear you telling them that their lunch is ready? The child is not ignoring you, they are simply too wrapped up in what they are doing to be distracted by anyone or anything. Put simply, meditation is me-time in its purest form.

Meditation should never be used as a substitute for medical treatment. Anyone who is suffering from clinical depression or any mild form of mental illness and anyone on any form of medication should first consult his (or her) doctor before beginning meditation.

Meditation is *not*:

- Self-hypnosis – which requires the participant to reach a state of semiconscious trance. Meditation is very much about the 'here and now' and its aim is to enable the meditator to 'live in the moment'.
- Relaxation – which is essentially passive, whereas meditation is an active focusing of the mind. While meditation attempts to transcend the normal thought processes, relaxation will often engage those very patterns of thought. However, meditation can be a great aid to relaxation, and relaxation a great aid to meditation.
- Necessarily tied to a religion – although meditation is used in all world religions, it does not specifically belong to any one nor is there any need for it to be tied to religion at all. Meditation can prove just as positive and spiritual an experience for an atheist as for a Buddhist.

- Concentration – which can be a means of achieving transcendence, but is not the object of the exercise. Concentrating on one thing is only a means to clearing the mind of all other thoughts. The object of your concentration is not important in itself, and, in fact, many meditators choose deliberately meaningless words or objects on which to concentrate for this very reason.

Meditation, frequently prescribed by holistic doctors, now has a stack of scientific evidence proving its enormous benefits to physical health. Those who meditate regularly believe that it leads to a significant lowering of tension and negative emotions, while at the same time deepening their sense of inner calm. This feeling of wellbeing brings physical benefits, for regular meditation eliminates or reduces stress, and in reducing stress, meditation can ease migraine and tension headaches, reduce blood pressure, benefit the heart and help to control pain.

Meditation can also be used for pain management and some people use the pain as a focus for their meditation, first locating and feeling it in all its intensity, and then picturing it as an entity that is something distinct from their inner self. This way the pain can be felt to be not intrinsic to that person, not as strong as the person, and conquerable by the person. As well as benefiting the sufferer in easing his (or her) discomfort, meditation can also be very empowering.

The need for a teacher

Like all things worth doing, the best way to learn meditation is to study with someone who has already mastered it. A good teacher should be qualified, compassionate, expert, patient, sincere and sympathetic, and someone in whom the pupil has complete confidence. Whether you are religious or not, a good person to guide you in the ways of meditation is an established religious

teacher, such as a rabbi or a priest. Apart from religious teachers, there are also qualified therapists.

Some people will prefer not to have a teacher at all, or be
unable to find someone suitable. Instead they might take their
instruction from books, lectures, courses and retreats. There are
a great number of religious books, from all faiths, that teach the
art of meditation. There are also many audio and visual tapes on
the market, aimed at the increasing numbers of people who are
turning to meditation either for health or spiritual reasons.

Regularly practising meditation combined with suitable yoga
postures and breathing exercises will induce a more positive
frame of mind throughout daily life as well as helping to release
tension and stress and alleviate pain. Before looking at the act
of meditation in more detail, the next section takes a brief look
at yoga and the role it can play in terms of your 'posture' or the
position you choose to adopt when meditating as well as its own
role in preventing headaches especially those caused by neck
tension.

Yoga

Stop what you are doing. Stand up, take a deep breath and have
a really good stretch. Standing on tiptoes, make yourself as tall
as possible with your hands reaching up to the sky and your
fingers splayed. Breathe out slowly, and slowly resume your normal standing posture. Now doesn't that feel good? Can you feel
the blood tingling in your hands and feet? Do the muscles in
your arms and legs feel relaxed and yet energised? Does your
mind, be it only for a fleeting moment, seem to have taken a
breather from its daily round of thoughts and worries? If your
answer is yes, then you are feeling the benefits of yoga already.

Yoga is a system of exercises designed to instil a sense of tran-
quillity and wellbeing in the practitioner. Its origins are lost in the
mists of time, though estimates suggest that it has been practised

in India for over 5,000 years. Hatha yoga, in particular, teaches techniques of physical control of the body through postures known as 'asanas' and breathing techniques called 'pranayama'. The asanas make the body supple and benefit the neuromuscular system, each posture combining mental acuity with breathing techniques and a specific body movement. Pranayama builds up the body's energy.

Yoga postures release tension in the neck and shoulders, increase circulation to the head, stimulate the nervous system and help alleviate pain ; yoga breathing exercises calm the mind and reduce stress and anxiety. A daily yoga session can help to prevent tension headaches and some postures can help to alleviate a headache that has already started. As with meditation, a good teacher is invaluable and will be able to suggest the correct poses to encourage the prevention of headaches as well as those which can alleviate pain once a headache is underway.

Yoga breathing

Yoga breathing is called pranayama. *Prana* means 'breath of life' and *ayama* means 'interval' so combined it means 'the interruption of breath'. The way that we breathe is inextricably linked to our sense of wellbeing and our emotions. When we are frightened or very stressed we start to take very quick, shallow breaths and when we are very relaxed, or asleep, our breathing becomes much slower and deeper. Both these processes are entirely involuntary, caused by the body reacting to signals sent out by the brain. Shallow breathing, while doing us no harm if sustained only for a short period, means that we are using only a fraction of the lungs' capacity, and failing to supply our muscles and organs, via the blood, with sufficient quantities of fresh oxygen. This results in those muscles and organs being unable to function properly.

Try taking a really deep breath right now. Do you feel as if you are taking in a lot more air than usual? And do you suddenly feel more alert than you did a moment ago? The fact is, lack of oxygen in the blood stream makes us feel tired and prone to headaches. Thus when we feel tired, we yawn. A yawn is the body's way of sucking in more air, just as a thermostat triggers an extra burst of energy in a heating system when the temperature falls below the set level.

Correct breathing can make a huge difference to the way we feel. A few deep breaths can help to ease off a mild case of indigestion. It can wake us up and help us to sleep. Recently it has been discovered that learning to play the bagpipes, which requires a great deal of deep breathing to generate enough air, can help to alleviate asthma. This is because the practice of deep breathing increases lung capacity and thereby helps the sufferer to take control of, rather than be controlled by, their breathing patterns.

Diaphragm breathing

To fully benefit from any yoga or meditation exercise it is helpful to breathe properly using the diaphragm as opposed to the chest. The diaphragm is the long flat muscle situated at the bottom of your lungs. To locate it, place your hand on your stomach, just below your ribs, and cough. You will feel a muscle tremble underneath your hand: this is your diaphragm. Now, keeping your hand where it is, repeat that coughing action slowly, but this time without restricting the flow of air from your throat, which you do when you cough. You will feel that a column of air is being pushed up through your body and that your diaphragm is contracting as it rises in accordance. Inhale deeply and you will feel the diaphragm expand as it lowers. Try holding a dictionary, or similar weight object, above your head. As you breathe you will be able to feel the diaphragm rising and falling. Focus on breathing using this muscle alone, remembering to keep your chest in and your shoulders down.

Opera singers and wind instrument musicians are well aware of the power of diaphragm breathing. Without it they would not be able to produce long, pure notes with their voices or control the volume and purity of sound from, for example, a clarinet. Short, weak breaths produce only warbling songs and ghastly clarinet squeaks! Next time you watch one of the world's great tenors perform, note how his chest does not rise or fall with his voice; the air that is powering his voice is being pumped up by his diaphragm.

Breathing in this way stimulates the solar plexus, the network of nerves that supply the abdominal area which is situated in what we refer to as the 'pit of the stomach'. A good supply of oxygen to this area will keep the inner organs, such as the kidneys and pancreas, functioning efficiently, which is clearly good for all-over health. It is this area that we refer to when we talk about a 'gut feeling', an instinct so strong that we feel it as opposed to just thinking it, and therefore tend to trust it more. Good yogic breathing will help to sharpen up your instincts too.

Diaphragm breathing requires a lot of practise in order to be able to do it without thinking. You do not need to restrict your practise of it to yoga sessions. Try doing it at odd moments throughout the day, until it becomes second nature.

Yoga postures for meditation

A short guide follows for some of the simple postures or asanas used when meditating. Do not expect to be able to do them at the first attempt and pay particular attention to the sequence of warm-up exercises. Even though yoga seems like a gentle exercise, it gives your muscles a serious workout. If you are at all unsure about the wisdom of attempting anything vis-a-vis your state of health it is imperative that you seek the advice of your doctor.

The first time you try some of these asanas you may find them uncomfortable. If so, do not force yourself to hold them for any length of time. Hard as it may be to believe, these postures will, with practice, one day come to seem very comfortable.

186

Before you begin, it is important:

- To establish a convenient, regular time to practise yoga and meditation.
- Not to have a full stomach.
- To wear comfortable and loose clothing.
- To use a clean, soft blanket or mat, thick enough to protect your spine and fit the length of your body.
- To perform each posture slowly, carefully and mindfully. Force and strain must be avoided.

Warm-up exercises

It is vital to begin any yoga session with this basic warm-up routine of simple movements.

1) Begin by waking up your feet by standing on tiptoe a couple of times, then returning them flat to the floor. Give your toes a good wriggle to get the blood moving and then stand with your feet together and your spine straight. To stand in the mountain posture, keep your knees loose by concentrating on lifting the muscles above them. Check that your abdomen is straight, not bulging out or curving in, and tuck in your buttocks. Let your hands, palms in, rest on the sides of your thighs. Take a deep breath and relax your shoulders and open your chest. Imagine a string from the crown of your head to the ceiling, and allow your facial muscles to relax. Breathe naturally and feel how the body maintains its balance, feel the space around you and the floor under your feet. This is best done with your eyes closed.

2) Standing in the mountain posture, keep your face forward, your feet together, your spine straight and your knees loose. Take a deep breath and as you exhale, slowly tilt your head to the left, your ear towards your

shoulder. As you breathe in , raise your head back into the centre and tilt to the right as you exhale. Repeat six times for each side. Concentrate on keeping these movements fluid and even. Now lower your chin to your chest as you exhale, raising it as you inhale. Repeat three times, then lower your head backwards as you breathe out and return to the upright position as you inhale.

3) Now lift both your shoulders up and back in a gentle backward rotation as if you were describing a small circle in the air. Try to keep these circles as perfect as possible. Do this five times then repeat this exercise in a forward motion, again five times. Both 2) and 3) are good exercises for releasing tension in the neck and shoulders throughout the day, something those who work at computers are particularly prone to.

4) Remaining in the mountain position, raise your hands above your head. Keep your arms parallel and intertwine your fingers so that your hands form a bridge. Still facing forward, stretch your arms up fully while keeping your feet flat on the ground. This will give your spine a good stretch.

5) Now return your left arm to your side, resting it palm downward on the side of your left thigh, keeping your right hand raised. Allow the right arm to lead you into a sideways stretch to the left. Keep your hips and chest facing forward and your feet flat. Now do a stretch to the right, leading with your raised left arm. Repeat three times on each side.

6) Allow your arms to hang loosely by your sides and swing gently to the left and then to the right in one slow movement. Keep your hips and chest facing forward and your feet flat, but allow your head and shoulders to move with the swing. Repeat three times.

7) Now for a back stretch. Fold your arms behind your back, holding each elbow with the opposite hand. If this

is too much of a strain, place both hands on the small of the back. Holding your hands firmly, tuck in your buttocks, push your hips out and your head and shoulders back so that your body forms a backward curve. Your weight should be centred on your heels. At first you may find this uncomfortably precarious, in which case you may want to hold onto the back of a chair to steady yourself. Do not, however, transfer any of your weight from your heels as you may topple over backwards.

8) For the forward stretch, keep your arms folded behind you or resting on the small of your back, and lean forwards towards the ground. Bend from the hips, keeping your back straight and your chin forward, until your torso forms a right angle with your legs. If you need a chair for balance, keep your hands on the back of the chair and gently step backwards until your back is straight. Stop the instant this becomes a strain, even if you feel that you have barely altered your position from the upright. Even the tiniest stretch is a step in the right direction.

9) Now for the legs. This exercise often requires the support of the back of a chair, which should be positioned by your right side. Facing forward, raise your right arm or hold the chair-back, and bend your left leg so that your heel reaches your right buttock. Grip the ankle with your left hand and hold. Ideally the left knee should be facing downwards. Hold for a short period, or until it becomes uncomfortable, then repeat for the opposite leg.

10) Repeat steps 4) and 5). Then give your legs and then your arms a gentle shake.

A beginner's posture for yoga and meditation

Lay out your blanket or mat, ensure that you are wearing nothing that is constricting, and begin by sitting down cross-legged. If this is too much of a strain on your thighs then prop up each knee with a cushion. Feeling uncomfortable will only sabotage your chances of relaxing. If this is still a strain, stretch your legs out in front of your body, about shoulders' width apart, with knees bent. You might want the further support of a folded-up blanket to sit on. Try not to be disheartened by difficulties, as your aches and pains will begin to ease up.

Make sure that your weight is not resting on the base of your spine but on your pelvic bone. The shape of your abdomen will tell you if you are sitting correctly, as it should be long and straight, not squashed and curved inwards. Straighten your back, lift your head and relax your shoulders. Imagine that there is a piece of string attached to the crown of your head, lifting it slightly towards the ceiling, but not so much that your spine 'locks' – you are not on military parade. Place your hands, palms upward, lightly upon your knees. Take a deep breath and exhale slowly. As you breathe try to focus on your body and how it feels. Let your shoulders rise and fall naturally with your breath.

Now imagine that each intake of breath as clean, white light and each outward breath as grey and smoky. Think of the white light as forcing out the tensions that have gathered inside you during the day; breathe out the stresses of the day and breathe in a mountain stream.

Allow yourself as long as you need to thoroughly focus on what you are doing, where you are and how your body feels. This is your very own time; allow yourself to sink into it. The world can wait. Once you are relaxed, give your arms a little stretch and slowly stand up.

Kneeling: the thunderbolt or the Japanese posture

This is the most basic sitting position. Simply kneel on the floor, keeping the knees together. Part the heels and bring the toes together so that you are sitting, straight-backed, on the insides of the feet with the hands on the knees. It is an excellent posture for breathing exercises, as well as for improving digestion and toning the thighs and spine. It is also surprisingly absorbing as it requires concentration to keep the spine and head erect and resist the impulse to slouch backwards. Sitting too erect is also damaging, as in so doing you contract the lower back thus making the spine feel stiff, resulting in its becoming less flexible. Interestingly this is the sitting pose adopted by participants in Japanese formal tea ceremonies that can last up to 5 hours, which just goes to show how comfortable and beneficial this posture can be.

Sitting: the sitting position or the Egyptian posture

If the thunderbolt is not at all comfortable, and you are sure that this is not down to following the instructions incorrectly, try the Egyptian posture. For this you need a firm chair with an upright back, and of sufficient height to allow your feet to be flat on the floor with your lower legs at right angles to your thighs. Think of the ancient Egyptian statues of kings and queens; they are serene and perfectly poised. This posture is identical. Keep your back and head erect; your chin should not jut out further than your forehead, and your abdomen should be long and straight, not squashed. Like the thunderbolt position, this will become enormously comfortable and, after a while, it will come to affect the way you sit outwith your yoga sessions – which is good news for the health of your spine as well as your posture.

Take care when getting in and out of this position. All too often, when we sit down on a chair we fall into it, rather than lower ourselves slowly downwards. The result of the former habit is that we make contact with the chair too heavily, some-times causing jarring, and, when it is time to get up, we do the opposite, and swing up from the seat, causing uneven and unnecessary strain throughout the whole body. A good way of changing your habits is to practise sitting on an imaginary chair. Notice how you lower yourself down gradually when you know that there is nothing to break your fall, and how you gently tilt your back forward from the hips, keeping it in alignment with the head. As you raise yourself up again, note how you gradually straighten your whole body, with your legs, head and spine working in harmony. Now try this with a real chair.

Lying flat: the corpse posture

You can take up this position for a meditation session or as a means of relaxing for a short time.

Begin by lying on your back. Lie flat on the floor on a carpet, blanket or hard mattress. Part the legs a little and let the feet flop to the side. The arms should be slightly away from the body, hands on the floor, palms up. Ensure that you are neither too hot nor too cold and that you are as comfortable as you can be. Now visualise yourself lying on a warm beach. Take a deep breath and feel the sun on your face and let your muscles relax into the soft sand. Allow yourself to breathe normally and enjoy the moment. When you are ready, bring your mind's focus down to your toes. Give them a little wiggle and then flex them. As they relax you will feel a great release of tension. Now move to the soles of your feet and flex and relax them as you did for your toes. Let your heels be heavy in the sand. Remember not to strain, and to perform the exercise slowly. Move up through your legs, tensing and relaxing your knees and then your buttocks. Take your internal gaze to your hands then move up your arms to your shoulders. Lift and flex your shoulders a couple of inches from the ground, and then sink back slowly as your relax. Tense and relax your facial muscles then allow them to soften. When you are completely relaxed lie still for a few minutes, simply concentrating on your breathing before starting your meditation proper. Give yourself a few moments to come out of this posture by focusing on where you are before you open your eyes.

Cupping the hands

Some teachers recommend that the hands be cupped if the pupil is in a posture where it is appropriate to do so. Right-handed people who decide to do this should cup the left hand over the right and, similarly, left-handed pupils should cup the right hand over the left, the point being to immobilise the dominant hand.

The meditation session

Once you are sitting comfortably in one of the yoga postures, spend a minute or two settling your body and mind, deciding which meditation you will do and how long you will meditate. Now run through your thoughts. Set your goals. Why are you about to meditate? What do you hope to achieve by it? The more motivated you are and the clearer your goal, the more successful the meditation is likely to be.

Which meditation technique?

There are many different meditation techniques and some are described in more detail in the pages that follow (*see* page 196). Some have been handed down from generation to generation for thousands of years and remain in their pure form. Others have been adapted to suit current circumstances. Deciding which of them is right for you can be quite bewildering, but bear in mind that the techniques are not ends in themselves: they are the motorway on which the journey to meditation moves. The best technique for you is the one with which you feel most comfortable.

The time and the place

There are no set rules as to how often you should meditate – some people meditate every day, others find just once a week suits them. Some people greatly enjoy meditation in the morning, just as the day is beginning. Others prefer the evening, because they can look forward to it during the day, and it helps them to relax and throw off their working cares, and therefore fully enjoy their evening.

If possible, set aside a corner of a suitable room for your meditation session. Make sure the area is clean, quiet and as pleasing as you can make it so that it is somewhere you will look forward to being in. Make sure, too, that you tell your family you don't want to be disturbed while you are meditating.

The atmosphere can be enhanced with sound: you could play a cassette of natural sounds such as the sea or bird song or Gregorian chants, and soft, indirect lighting is very comforting. Colours too are also important: bright red will keep you alert but also distract you from your meditation, a gentle blue or white will match your calm. Some people burn candles and incense sticks. If you think they will help you to meditate or make the room more conducive to meditation by all means follow their example. Remember that to meditate effectively you must be as relaxed as possible.

The meditation object

This is something on which the attention can focus and on which it may rest, ideally for the full session, although in practice this rarely happens as even experienced meditators may find their attention wandering at some time or other (*see* **Common Problems** below), but the meditation object is always there to come back to.

The object may be something to look at – a flower, a candle, a religious icon or a mandala or yantra (symbols specially designed for meditation). It may be something you can listen to – a recording of the sound of the sea or a running river or bird song, for example. It can be as everyday as the ticking of the clock or as esoteric as the tinkling of temple bells.

Many meditators use a mantra – a word or phrase repeated again and again either out loud or mentally (see page 204). The meditation object can even be your own breathing.

Common problems

Even the most practised meditators may experience difficulties, so beginners should not be put off if they find it hard to get into a meditative state of mind or to maintain concentration. One of the most common problems is mental excitement. The mind becomes restless and the attention is continually distracted. Sometimes we are unable to banish nagging problems from our thoughts – for example, job security, paying household bills, health worries. If you are in a particularly good frame of mind, you may unintentionally recall things that have made you smile – a new friendship, an enjoyable conversation, even a television programme we have enjoyed.

In our everyday lives we let our minds jump from thought to thought, from worry to worry, so mental wandering is a deeply ingrained habit and, like any habit, is difficult to give up. One popular way of overcoming it is to concentrate on breathing, which has a very calming effect on your state of mind. Be patient. It takes time and practice to learn how to slow and control the mind. Don't give up.

Another common problem is drowsiness. When we are in a completely relaxed frame of mind, it is all too easy to drop off. If you start to feel sleepy while meditating, make sure that you are sitting up straight and your head is not bent too far forward. If you are meditating with your eyes closed, open them and meditate with the gaze directed at the floor just in front of you. If you are meditating in a centrally heated room, turn down the heating or open a window to freshen the air. Increasing the amount of light in the room can also help you to stay awake.

Physical tension or pain can be resolved by focusing your attention for a moment on each part of the body in turn, starting with the head and working downwards, making a conscious effort to make it relax. You can do this at the start of the session or during it if need be. Deep, slow breathing can also help. Concentrate as hard as you can, and as you breathe out, try to imagine the pain or tension evaporating.

Breaking the spell

Avoid coming out of meditation too quickly, for if you do, most of the benefits you have achieved will be lost. Once you have finished meditating remain in your meditative position for a minute or two and then slowly stretch, catlike, quietly reflecting on how good you now feel – calmer and better equipped to cope with life.

Some meditation techniques

Breathing meditations

Awareness of breath meditation

Correct abdominal breathing lies at the heart of all kinds of meditation. In 'awareness of breath' meditation, breathing itself is the object of the meditation. Such meditation is held in the highest regard among Buddhists, Hindus and Taoists, all of whom believe in it not just as a means of inducing peace of mind but also of encouraging physical and mental health.

Breathing awareness can also be used as a prelude to a different form of meditation. If this is to be the case, 5 minutes or so will calm the nerves and focus and still the mind, putting it in a receptive mood for the session proper.

Awareness of breath meditation techniques are ideal for the novice meditator because they are entirely natural and most people feel quite comfortable with them. The techniques simply involve being aware of the breath as it enters and leaves the body.

Sit motionless in any of the postures you find comfortable, remembering to keep the back, head and neck in perfect balance, and begin to think about your breathing, becoming aware of each intake of breath, the pause, the expulsion of stale air from the lungs, the pause, the next breath. Your attention will wander. Don't be put off; bring it back to the object of your meditation and start again on the next inhalation.

It is not unusual for the pattern of breathing to change during meditation. At first, when you may be feeling a little self-conscious, you may find that you are holding each breath for longer than usual, but as the meditation proceeds you should find that breathing becomes smoother and deeper, or it may become shallow and slow. Don't be concerned by this. As you concentrate on your breathing and lose yourself in the meditation, the body establishes a rate of breathing that is right for that particular time.

There are several methods for encouraging attention to focus on the breath. None of them is better than any of the others. Try them all, and if you are happier with one over the rest, stick with it. Naturally they all require you to adopt a suitable posture and choose an appropriate place. The simplest method involves taking up a comfortable posture, shutting your eyes to aid concentration, although it is better to keep them half open and breathing as naturally as you can, counting either each inhalation or exhalation up to 10. Repeat this for 20 minutes. Counting is an aid to concentration and helps to prevent the mind from wandering.

Some people find it helps if they focus their attention on the tip of the nose or the inside of the nostrils as the breath enters and leaves the body. Others use the movement of the abdomen as the focus of their attention.

Mindfulness of breathing meditation or 'following the breath'

'A monk having gone to the forest, to the foot of a tree, or to an empty place, sits down cross-legged, keeps his body erect and his mindfulness alert. Just mindful he breathes in and mindful he breathes out.' Thus did the Suddha advocate to his followers the mindfulness of breathing meditation.

According to this widely practised method of meditation, the abdomen or nose is the focus of attention, which is a development of the basic awareness of breath meditation which many people find unsatisfying after a month or so.

There is no counting in mindfulness of breath meditation; rather it is the flow of breath in and out on which the mind is concentrated. To practise it, sit comfortably in any of the prescribed positions with the eyes closed and breathe in and out quite naturally, focusing the attention either on the abdomen or the nose.

If focusing on the abdomen, become aware of the pause in breathing at the limit of each sea-swell-like rise and fall of the abdomen. If focusing on the nose, concentrate on the nostrils where the flow of inhaled and exhaled air can be felt.

You are certain to find at first that your attention wanders even if you have been successfully practising counting the breath meditation for some time. When you realise that your attention has meandered, simply return it to the abdomen or nose and continue the meditation.

As you give in to the seductive rhythm of your abdomen as it rises and falls or your sensation of the inflow or outflow of air in the nostrils, your breathing will become smoother and much quieter as the meditation deepens.

Try to avoid controlling your breathing in any way. This can be difficult. Watching the breath without trying to interfere with it seems simple, but it takes some practice for the mind to become used to the fact that you are trying to surrender yourself completely to the spontaneous flow of the breath. Beginners usually find that their breathing becomes uneven, quickening and slowing for no apparent reason. They should not worry, for in time the breath settles to its own rhythm.

Many of those who practise following the breath meditation find it helps if they make themselves aware of the journey of each breath from the moment it enters the nostril to the moment it is expelled. Others picture an aura of energy and light just in front of the forehead. With each breath some of the power is taken into the body and the meditator focuses on its journey deep into the body.

Sensory awareness meditation

Movement is also a part of this sensory awareness meditation in which it is combined with breathing awareness.

Begin by lying on your back on a rug or mat. Your legs can be fully extended or drawn in towards the buttocks with the feet flat on the floor. When you are comfortable, close your eyes and concentrate for a few minutes on letting each part of the body in turn sink more deeply into the floor, starting with the feet and moving upwards through the calves, knees, thighs, pelvis, rib cage, chest, hands, lower arms, elbows, upper arms and neck to the head. Concentrate not just on the surfaces that are in contact with the floor but with the sides and top too.

Now, concentrating on each exhalation of breath, try to feel your whole body sink deeply into the floor.

After about 15 minutes, lay the hands on the diaphragm, keeping the upper arms and elbows firmly on the floor. After the diaphragm has moved the hands up and down, up and down for a minute or two, they will feel as if they have been incorporated into the breathing process. Very slowly raise them a little from the body, concentrating all the time on your breathing, then return them to the diaphragm, allowing them once again to become part of the breathing process.

Repeat this for 10 minutes or so, gradually increasing the distance the hands are moved away from the body each time until they eventually come to land on the floor. Slowly you will come to think that the whole cycle is happening by itself with absolutely no effort on your part, and you will find yourself at one with the world.

Visual meditation

Tratek (gazing meditation)
Gazing meditation involves contemplating an object without judgement or thought, simply revelling in its existence. Choose

your object with care: you want something neither too complex nor with negative associations for you. If thoughts intrude upon your meditation, chase them away by renewing your attentions on your chosen object.

Place the object of your meditation at eye level between 1 and 2 metres from your face. If you decide to use a mandala or yantra the central point should be level with the eyes. Assume whichever meditation position you favour, and in as relaxed a way as possible, gaze at the image, focusing your attention on it, trying to become absorbed in what you are looking at rather than just thinking about it.

After 2 or 3 minutes or as soon as you feel any indication of eye strain, close your eyes and visualise the object for as long as you can, still attempting to be part of it. Open your eyes again and continue alternating open-eyed and closed-eyed meditation for the full session.

Initially it will be difficult to retain the image in your mind's eye for long when your eyes are closed: don't worry. When the image starts to fade, open the eyes and gaze at the object again. As you become more practised in the art, you will find that you can retain the image for longer and longer.

Meditating on a candle
Many of those who come to visual meditation for the first time find that a lighted candle in a darkened room is the ideal object of focus. This may be because we associate a candle flame with peace and enlightenment, and find it both a comforting and inspiring thing to gaze upon.

One method recommended for beginners is to light a candle in a darkened, draught-free room: draught-free so that the flame burns as steadily as possible. To meditate on a candle, sit as motionless as you can in any of the recommended positions and gaze at the flame so that it holds your attention completely. Do not analyse why this image fascinates you, or allow your mind to wander onto thoughts of the candle's heat or brightness: simply look. Let the image fill your mind for a minute before quickly closing the eyes. Notice how the candle has imprinted itself on the darkness. Hold it in your mind's eye, not worrying about any change of colour. If it slips to the side, bring it back to the centre and keep concentrating until the image fades completely. Now open the eyes and resume gazing at the candle. Continue in this way for 10 minutes at first, gradually increasing the time until you can sit comfortably for a full 20 minutes.

Purification visualising

Purification is a recurring theme in Buddhist meditation. When we see ourselves as impure or negative, that is what we become. With our self-esteem at a low ebb we feel limited and inadequate and don't give ourselves a chance to change. Believing that we are pure in essence is the first step to becoming pure in practice.

This simple meditation contains the essence of purification, banishing problems and mistakes, trying to see them as temporary intrusions, not as part of our nature.

Begin by settling comfortably into a suitable position, then concentrate on breathing normally and observing how long each exhalation and inhalation lasts. After a minute or two, imagine that all your negative energy, the mistakes you have made in the past, the things that are holding you back are leaving your body in a cloud of black smoke each time you breathe out. When you inhale, visualise that everything positive in the universe is entering your body in a stream of white light, as radiant as it is pure. Visualise it flowing to every part of your body, bathing it in its intensity.

Banish distractions by seeing them as black smoke and exhale them along with the other negative aspects of your experience.

Bubbles of thought meditation

Sitting in a comfortable position, visualise your mind as the smooth, calm surface of a pond. As thoughts enter your mind, see them as bubbles rising from the depths of the pond. They should be observed, not pursued, so that the conscious and deliberate following through of each thought is avoided and you become detached from it as you watch it bubble to the surface. Note the thought and then gently return to contemplating the smooth, rippleless surface of the pond.

As time passes and you pass into deeper layers of consciousness, see yourself sinking under the surface of the pond, becoming one with it. After about 10 minutes, refocus your mind on your surroundings to bring the meditation to a conclusion.

Sound meditation

Sounds have a profound effect upon us. They can stimulate deep emotions and even prompt physical responses. Some sounds prompt memories, the strain of a long-forgotten hymn can transport someone back to their schooldays, while the rattle of familiar keys in the lock can make a person feel reassured and happy. However, it is not all to do with memory. Beautiful music can move us to tears or uplift us so that we feel our heart 'soar' with the melody. The sound of waves breaking on a shore induces a sense of peace, while the rumble of thunder makes us alert, perhaps even very nervous. And our recall of sounds is generally much better than we realise. We can learn to recognise someone by the sound of their footsteps, and know instinctively when a sound is 'out of place', such as an unfamiliar creak on a floorboard or a false note in someone's voice.

Concentrating using sound is a viable alternative for anyone who finds visualisation difficult. In some cases, this latter is simply a case of being unable to concentrate fully and will improve with practice. For others, however, it will remain difficult, because the person has a better-developed aural memory than a visual one. A way of determining this is to imagine a tennis ball. Picture it, concentrating on its rough texture, its colour and its shape. Keep concentrating until that picture is fully in your mind. Now imagine you have thrown the tennis ball against a wall and it has bounced off and along the pavement. Can you hear it? If you find the listening substantially easier, and more absorbing, than the looking, you may want to try using sound rather than images.

Hamsa

Hamsa is a Sanskrit word meaning bird, and the hamsa meditation involves visualising a bird in flight. Take a few deep breaths and fill your mind with the image of a clear blue sky. Now picture a bird soaring across it, watch it swoop and soar across your field of vision. Take a deep breath and as you inhale say the word 'ham', and as you exhale, say 'sa'. Repeat this several times and just allow the bird to fly away, but keep visualising that sky. Keep up this gentle chanting for several minutes, and you will find that your mind has cleared itself of intruding thoughts and is absorbed by the blue and the notes of the chant.

Inner sounds (nadas)

Concentrating on inner sounds is another way of shutting out external sounds and thoughts. It also develops increased awareness of your own body and its internal workings. Begin by placing your fingers over your ears; this will shut out external noise. Close your eyes and allow your breathing to relax. As your mind becomes still you will become aware of a steady surging, rumbling sound. In fact, you will be amazed by the noise in there! Keep listening carefully, remembering to keep your body relaxed and your mind focused. Beneath this rumbling sound you will eventually discern subtler sounds. As they become apparent, hone your focus in towards them. If your mind begins to wander, switch back to the louder sounds, then back to the subtler ones behind them. Ultimately your mind will become absorbed by these quieter sounds and you will experience a deep sense of serenity. When you come out of this exercise you may feel surprised at how quiet the outside world is by comparison.

Don't be discouraged if, the first few times you try this, you hear only the surging sounds. Like all meditation techniques, it requires practice and patience.

Repeating a mantra

Repeating a word or phrase – 'a mantra' – over and over again is probably the most practised and widespread path to meditation and one of the oldest. Mantra yoga is mentioned in the Vedas, the oldest of the world's scriptures. The mantra may be chanted aloud or repeated silently. The repetition of the mantra is known in India as *japa*, and according to the traditions of that country there are fourteen different kinds of japa. Today, in the West, only two of them are in common use – voiced repetition and mental repetition.

The power of the mantra is the power of sound to affect people and alter their state of mind. If you doubt that sound can do this, pause for a moment and consider how irritated you get if someone is playing music too loudly or if you are sitting next to someone who is plugged into a personal stereo and the music is almost inaudible to you. If sound can irritate, then surely the converse is true – sound can make you feel tranquil – and to focus on a mantra during meditation can lead to some of the deepest and most profound sessions you are likely to experience.

Sound is energy produced by a vibrating object. We can hear waves within a certain frequency band, and we interpret different frequencies as different sounds. If the frequencies are above this band, they are called ultrasonic, if below, infrasonic. The body absorbs all frequencies, even the ones that the ear cannot hear, and they can have a profound effect upon us, even to the extent of altering our moods. This influence is now being utilised in some forms of therapy.

There is also the matter of resonance. This latter is the phenomena whereby one vibration can cause another, as, for example, someone singing a clear, high, sustained note might produce a ringing resonance in a crystal glass. Mantras are not arbitrary gatherings of words that sound pleasant, but deliberate constructions that utilise the phenomena of sound, frequency and resonance. Followers of mantra meditation believe that the mantra sounds resonate with different energy centres in the body. Most of the major religions have their own mantra but for those who wish to use a mantra in their meditation but who want to avoid religion, any word or phrase, no matter how meaningless, will do.

Those who are suspicious of any religious aspects associated with mantra can also choose their mantra by the method recommended by Lawrence LeShan, a leading expert in the subject. He advocates the 'la-de' method of mantra selection: simply opening a telephone directory at random and blindly letting the forefinger fall on the page. The first syllable of that name becomes the first syllable of the mantra. Repeat the process, linking the second syllable selected at random with the first and – hey presto – you have a mantra!

To practise meditation with a mantra, begin, as usual, by taking up the position that you find most comfortable and breathe gently and rhythmically through the nostrils, taking the breath deep into the abdomen. Then repeat the mantra, either aloud or silently inward, focusing your concentration on it as completely as you can. When your mind has become still, it is no longer necessary to continue repeating the mantra, but, as with other forms of meditation, when you become aware that your thoughts have wandered, start repeating the mantra again, concentrating your conscious thoughts on it.

Once you have chosen a mantra with which you are comfortable, stick with it. It is amazing how in times of stress, repeating your mantra a few times silently to yourself restores calm and helps you to put things into proper perspective.

Many mantra meditators repeat the mantra in rhythm with their breathing, saying it once or twice on inhalation and once or twice on breathing out. They are usually repeated silently, but some teachers encourage their pupils to say them aloud, especially if they are leading a group meditation.

Om

Om, a Sanskrit word pronounced to rhyme with 'Rome', is one of the most widely used mantras. According to Hindu belief, om is the primal sound and it is accorded the highest value as an object of meditation and is one well worth trying. Breathe in gently, and as you exhale recite the word as three sounds, 'a' (as in father), 'oo' (as in room) and 'mmm'. Try to feel the sounds vibrating in your body. The 'a' will feel as if it is ringing in your belly, the 'oo' will resonate in your chest and the 'mmm' will positively resound in the bones of your skull. Link the sounds to your breathing rhythm, keeping it slow and calm and avoiding deepening it in any way.

After saying 'om' aloud for 10 breaths, soften the voice until you are saying the word under your breath, then lower it even further, keeping your attention firmly focused on it. It won't be long before your lips stop moving and the syllables lose their shape, leaving you with just an idea that clings to your mind. Banish any intrusive thoughts by imagining them as puffs of smoke and watch them being blown away by a gentle breeze.

Music and meditation

The relevance of music as an aid to meditation is a personal one. Its effect depends on facilitating your meditations, and that in turn depends on your own instinct and intuition.

Percussion instruments have long been used in meditation, especially where it is practised by atavists. The music they produce symbolises rhythm and vitality.

Gongs and bells are said to purify the surrounding atmosphere making it more conducive to meditation. Many religions use peals of bells to help their adherents gather wandering thoughts.

If you want to use bells as an aid to meditation, focus your thoughts on the sound, trying to experience it beyond audibility.

Harps have long been associated with meditation. In China the cheng and other zither-like instruments are widely used, while in India, the sitar and the vina accompany meditative chanting.

The gentle tinkling of the Aeolian harp can create a perfectly calm state of mind as you approach your meditations and help to focus your thoughts.

To meditate to music, take up your usual position, close your eyes and listen to a favourite piece, immersing yourself in it completely. Try to become one with the music, letting the sound encompass you. If you find that your thoughts are invaded by memories associated with the piece that you have selected, imagine them as musical notes floating off into the distance.

Tactile meditation

Before you begin, choose an object to hold while you are meditating – something light, for if it is too heavy its weight will affect your concentration and hence your ability to focus on it. It need not be particularly soft, but it should not be sharp. Now close your eyes and concentrate on the texture of the object in your hand, focusing on how it feels rather than on what it is.

Another method of using touch to help reach the meditative state requires either a set of worry beads or four or five pebbles. Relax in your favourite position, holding the beads or pebbles in the open palm of one hand and with the other move them rhythmically and methodically between your fingers, counting them one at a time. Feel each bead or pebble as you count, focusing all your attention on the slow, repetitive movement.

Chapter 24

OSTEOPATHY

What is osteopathy?

Osteopathy is a treatment that uses manipulation and massage to help distressed muscles and joints and make them work smoothly.

The profession began in 1892 when Dr Andrew Taylor Still (1828–1917), an American farmer, inventor and doctor, opened the USA's first school of osteopathic medicine. He sought alternatives to the medical treatments of his day which he believed were ineffective as well as often harmful.

Still's new philosophy of medicine, based upon the teachings of Hippocrates, advocated that 'Finding health should be the purpose of a doctor. Anyone can find disease.' Like Hippocrates, Still recognised that the human body is a unit in which structure, function, mind and spirit all work together. Osteopathic therapy aims to pinpoint and treat any problems that are of a mechanical nature. The body's frame consists of the skeleton, muscles, joints and ligaments and all movements or activities such as running, swimming, eating, speaking and walking depend upon it.

Still came to believe that it would be safer to encourage the body to heal itself, rather than use the drugs that were then available but that were not always safe. He regarded the body from an engineer's point of view and the combination of this and his medical experience of anatomy, led him to believe that ailments and disorders could occur when the bones or joints no longer functioned in harmony. He believed that manipulation was the cure for the problem. Although his ideas provoked a great deal of opposition from the American medical profession at first, they slowly came to be accepted. The bulk of scientific research has been done in America with a number of medical schools of osteopathy being established. Dr Martin Littlejohn, who was a pupil of Dr Still, brought the practice of osteopathy to the UK around 1900, with the first school being founded in 1917 in London. He emphasised the compassionate care and treatment of the person as a whole, not as a collection of symptoms or unrelated parts. The philosophy and practices of A. T. Still, considered radical in the 1800s, are generally accepted principles of good medicine today.

Treatment

Problems that prevent the body from working correctly or create pain can be due to an injury or stress. For example, stress can cause a contraction in the muscles situated at the back of the neck and at the base of the skull which can result in a tension headache. Some relief can be obtained by the use of massage.

The majority of an osteopath's patients suffer from disorders of the spine, which result in pain in the lower part of the back and the neck. A great deal of pressure is exerted on the spinal column, and especially on the cartilage between the individual vertebrae. This is a constant pressure due to the effects of gravity that occurs merely by standing. If a person stands incorrectly with stooped shoulders, this will exacerbate any problems or perhaps initiate one. In osteopathy, it is believed that if the basic framework of the body is undamaged, then all physical activities can be accomplished efficiently and without causing any problems, so the joints and framework of the body are manipulated and massaged where necessary so that the usual action is regained. Athletes or dancers can receive injuries to muscles or joints such as the ankle, hip, wrist or elbow and they too can benefit from treatment by osteopathy. Pain in the lower back can be experienced by pregnant women who may stand in a different way due to their increasing weight and, if this is the case, osteopathy can often ease matters considerably.

Another form of therapy, known as *cranial osteopathy*, can be used for patients suffering from pain in the face or head. This is effected by the osteopath using slight pressure on these areas including the upper part of the neck. (*See* **Cranial Osteopathy** on page 159.)

To find a fully qualified osteopath, it is advisable to contact the relevant professional body, or your GP may be able to help. It is now common practice for doctors to recommend osteopathy to some patients and some GPs use the therapy themselves after receiving training. Although its benefits are generally accepted for problems of a mechanical nature, it is vital that your doctor first decides what is wrong before any possible use can be made of osteopathy.

The first visit

At the first visit to an osteopath, he (or she) will need to know the complete history of any problems experienced, how they first occurred and what eases or aggravates matters. A patient's case history and any form of therapy that is currently in use will all be of relevance to the practitioner. A thorough examination will then take place observing how the patient sits, stands or lies down and also the manner in which the body is bent to the side, back or front. As each movement takes place, the osteopath is able to take note of the extent and ability of the joint to function. The practitioner will also feel the muscles, soft tissues and ligaments to detect if there is any tension present. Whilst examining the body, the osteopath will note any problems that are present and, as an aid to diagnosis, use may also be made of checking reflexes, such as the kneejerk reflex. If a patient has been involved in an accident, X-rays can be checked to determine the extent of any problem. It is possible that a disorder may not benefit from treatment by osteopathy and the patient would be advised accordingly. If this is not the case, treatment can commence with the chosen course of therapy.

Consultations – how long and how many?

Patients generally find that each consultation is quite pleasant and they feel much more relaxed and calm afterwards. The length of each session can vary, but it is generally in the region of half an hour. As the osteopath gently manipulates the joint, it will lessen any tenseness present in the muscles and also improve its ability to work correctly and to its maximum extent. It is this manipulation that can cause a clicking noise to be heard. As well as manipulation, other methods such as massage can be used to good effect. Muscles can be freed from tension if the tissue is massaged and this will also stimulate the flow of blood. In some cases, the patient may experience a temporary deterioration once treatment has commenced, and this is more likely to occur if the ailment has existed for quite some time.

There is no set number of consultations necessary, as this will depend upon the nature of the problem and also for how long it has been apparent. It is possible that a severe disorder that has arisen suddenly can be alleviated at once. The osteopath is likely to recommend a number of things so that patients can help themselves between treatments. Techniques such as learning to relax, how to stand and sit correctly and additional exercises can be suggested by the osteopath.

Driving – the osteopathic way

People who have to spend a lot of their life driving are susceptible to a number of problems related to the manner in which they are seated. If their position is incorrect they can suffer from tension headaches, pain in the back, and the shoulders and neck can feel stiff. There are a number of ways in which these problems can be remedied such as holding the wheel in the approved manner at roughly 10 to 2 on the dial of a clock. The arms should not be held out straight and stiff, but should feel relaxed and be bent at the elbow. In order that the driver can maintain a position in which the back and neck feel comfortable, the seat should be moved so that it is tilting backwards a little, although it should not be so far away that the pedals are not easily reached. The legs should not be held straight out, and if the pedals are the correct distance away the knees should be bent a little and feel quite comfortable. It is also important to sit erect and not slump in the seat. The driver's rear should be positioned right at the back of the seat and this should be checked each time before using the vehicle. It is also important that there is adequate vision from the mirror so its position should be altered if necessary. If the driver already has a back problem then it is a simple matter to provide support for the lower part of the back. If this is done it should prevent strain on the shoulders and backbone.

Whilst driving, the person should make a conscious effort to ensure that the shoulders are not tensed, but held in a relaxed way. Another point to remember is that the chin should not be stuck out but kept in, otherwise the neck muscles will become tensed and painful. Drivers can perform some beneficial exercises while they are waiting in a queue of traffic. To stretch your neck muscles, put the chin right down on to the chest and then relax. This stretching exercise should be done several times. Contracting and relaxing the muscles of the stomach can also be done at the same time as driving and will have a positive effect on the flow of blood to the legs and also will improve how you are seated. Another exercise involves raising your shoulders upwards and then moving them backwards in a circular motion. Your head should also be inclined forward a little. This should also be done several times to gain the maximum effect.

Chapter 25

REFLEXOLOGY

What is reflexology?

Reflexology is a technique of diagnosis and treatment in which certain areas of the body, particularly the feet, are massaged to alleviate pain or other symptoms in the organs of the body. It is thought to have originated about five thousand years ago in China and was also used by the ancient Egyptians. It was introduced to Western society by Dr William Fitzgerald, who was an ear, nose and throat consultant in America. He applied 10 zones (or energy channels) to the surface of the body, hence the term 'zone therapy', and these zones, or channels, were considered to be paths along which flowed a person's vital energy, or 'energy force'. The zones ended at the hands and feet. Thus, when pain was experienced in one part of the body, it could be relieved by applying pressure elsewhere in the body, within the same zone.

Subsequent practitioners of reflexology have concentrated primarily on the feet, although the working of reflexes throughout the body can be employed to beneficial effect.

Treatment

Reflexology uses a specific type of massage at the correct locations on the body. The body's energy flow is thought to follow certain routes, connecting every organ and gland with an ending or pressure point on the feet, hands or another part of the body. When the available routes are blocked, and a tenderness on the body points to such a closure, then it indicates some ailment or condition in the body that may be somewhere other than the tender area. The massaging of particular reflex points enables these channels to be cleared, restoring the energy flow and at the same time healing any damage.

The uses of reflexology are numerous, and it is especially effective for the relief of pain (headaches, back pain and toothache), treatment of digestive disorders, stress and tension, colds and influenza, asthma, arthritis, and more. It is also possible to predict a potential illness and either give preventive therapy or suggest that specialist advice be sought. The massaging action of reflexology creates a soothing effect that enhances blood flow, to the overall benefit of the whole body. (Reflexology, however, clearly cannot be used to treat conditions that require surgery.)

Reflex massage initiates a soothing effect to bring muscular and nervous relief while the pressure of a finger applied to a particular point (or nerve ending) may create a sensation elsewhere in the body, indicating the connection or flow between the two points. Although pain may not be alleviated immediately, continued massage over periods of up to an hour will usually have a beneficial effect.

Some practitioners believe that stimulation of the reflex points leads to the release of endorphins (in a manner similar to acupuncture). Endorphins are compounds that occur in the brain and have pain-relieving qualities similar to those of morphine.

They are derived from a substance in the pituitary gland and are involved in endocrine control (glands producing hormones, for example, the pancreas, thyroid, ovary and testis).

The best way to undergo reflexology is in the hands of a therapist, who will usually massage all reflex areas, concentrating on any tender areas that will correspond to a part of the body that is ailing. Although there have not been any clinical trials to ascertain the efficacy of reflexology, it is generally thought that it does little harm and, indeed, much benefit may result.

There are certain conditions for which reflexology is inappropriate, including diabetes, some heart disorders, osteoporosis, disorders of the thyroid gland, and phlebitis (inflammation of the veins). It may also not be suitable for pregnant women or anyone suffering from arthritis of the feet.

Chapter 26

SHIATSU

What is shiatsu?

Shiatsu originated in China at least two thousand years ago, when the earliest accounts gave the causes of ailments and the remedies that could be effected through a change of diet and way of life. The use of massage and acupuncture was also recommended. The Japanese also practised this massage, after it had been introduced into their country, and it was known as *anma*. The therapy that is known today as shiatsu has gradually evolved with time from anma under influences from both East and West. It is only very recently that it has gained recognition and popularity, with people becoming aware of its existence and benefits.

Although East and West have different viewpoints on health and life, these can complement one another. The Eastern belief is of a primary flow of energy throughout the body, which runs along the channels known as meridians. It is also believed that this energy exists throughout the universe and that all living creatures are dependent upon it as much as on physical nourishment. The energy is known by three similar names, *ki, chi* and *prana* in Japan, China and India respectively. (It should be noted that the term 'energy' in this context is not the same as the physical quantity that is measured in joules or calories.) As in acupuncture, in shiatsu there are certain pressure points on the meridians that relate to certain organs, and these points are known as *tsubos*.

Treatment

Shiatsu is a relaxing treatment that uses hand pressure and manipulative techniques to adjust the body's physical structure and its natural inner energies in order to help ward off illness and maintain good health. Shiatsu can be used to treat a variety of problems such as headaches, insomnia, anxiety, back pain, etc. According to Chinese medicine, a headache is not just an event in the head, nor is it merely a pain or something to be stopped without regard for its origins, nor should it be treated on the same basis as someone else's headache. Rather, it is an obstruction of ki, related to the overall energy patterns in the whole body of the particular individual, their circumstances, and lifestyle. Treatment might involve work on the arms or legs as well as (or instead of) the head and will bring more lasting and satisfactory changes than will an attempt to block the superficial symptoms.

Western medicine may be unable to find a physical cause for a health problem, and although some pain relief may be provided, the underlying cause of the problem may not be cured. But it is possible that one session of shiatsu will be sufficient to remedy the problem by stimulating the flow of energy along the body's channels or meridians. A regime of exercise (possibly a specific routine) with a change in diet and/or lifestyle may also be recommended. Shiatsu can encourage a general feeling of good health in the whole person, not just in the physical sense. There are many benefits for both the giver and the receiver of shiatsu on a physical and a spiritual level.

Appendix
USEFUL ORGANISATIONS

USEFUL ORGANISATIONS

The Migraine Action Association
27 East Street
Leicester
LE1 6NB
Tel: 0116 275 8317
Fax: 0116 254 2023
E-mail: info@migraine.org.uk
www.migraine.org.uk

The Migraine Trust
52-53 Russell Square
London
WC1B 4HP
Tel: 020 7631 6970
Fax: 020 7436 2886
Email: info@migrainetrust.org
www.migrainetrust.org

M.A.G.N.U.M. (US)
The National Migraine Association
www.migraines.org

MIDAS
www.midas-migraine.net

Headache Care Center (US)
www.headachecare.com

The Organisation for the Understanding of Cluster Headaches
www.clusterheadaches.com

The British Association for the Study of Headaches
www.bash.org.uk

The International Federation of Professional Aromatherapists
82 Ashby Road
Hinckley
Leicestershire
LE10 1SN
Tel: 01455 637987
www.ifparoma.org

The Society of Homeopaths
11 Brookfield
Duncan Close
Moulton Park
Northampton
NN3 6WL
Tel: 01604 817890
Fax: 01604 648848
E-mail: info@homeopathy-soh.org
www.homeopathy-soh.org

National Institute of Medical Herbalists
Clover House
James Court
South Street
Exeter
EX1 1EE
Tel: 01392 426022
E-mail: info@nimh.org.uk
www.nimh.org.uk

The British Acupuncture Council
www.acupuncture.org.uk

The British Reflexology Association
Administration Office
Monks Orchard
Whitbourne
Worcester
WR6 5RB
Tel: 01886 821207
E-mail: bra@britreflex.co.uk
www.britreflex.co.uk

The Institute of Osteopathy
3 Park Terrace
Manor Road
Luton
Bedfordshire
LU1 3HN
Tel: 01582 488455
Fax: 01582 481533
E-mail: enquiries@osteopathy.org
www.osteopathy.org

The Society of Teachers of the Alexander Technique (STAT)
1st Floor
Linton House
39–51 Highgate Road
London
NW5 1RT
Tel: 020 7482 5135
Fax: 020 7482 5435
E-mail: enquiries@stat.org.uk
www.stat.org.uk

Shiatsu Society UK
PO Box 4580
Rugby
Warwickshire
CV21 9EL.
Tel: 0845 130 4560
Fax: 01788 547111
www.shiatsusociety.org